CW00392695

THE METABOLIC APPROACH TO OBESITY 4.0
© Copyright 2022 by SCOTT J. BARNARD

This document is geared towards providing exact and reliable information with regards to the topic and issue covered. The publication is sold with the idea that the publisher is not required to render accounting, officially permitted, or otherwise, qualified services. If advice is necessary, legal or professional, a practiced individual in the profession should be ordered.

From a Declaration of Principles which was accepted and approved equally by a Committee of the American Bar Association and a Committee of Publishers and Associations.

In no way is it legal to reproduce, duplicate, or transmit any part of this document in either electronic means or in printed format. Recording of this publication is strictly prohibited and any storage of this document is not allowed unless with written permission from the publisher.

All rights reserved.

The information provided herein is stated to be truthful and consistent, in that any liability, in terms of inattention or otherwise, by any usage or abuse of any policies, processes, or directions contained within is the solitary and utter responsibility of the recipient reader. Under no circumstances will any legal responsibility or blame be held against the publisher for any reparation, damages, or monetary loss due to the information herein, either directly or indirectly.

Respective authors own all copyrights not held by the publisher.

The information herein is offered for informational purposes solely, and is universal as so.

The presentation of the information is without contract or any type of guarantee assurance.

The trademarks that are used are without any consent, and the publication of the trademark is without permission or backing by the trademark owner.

All trademarks and brands within this book are for clarifying purposes only and are the owned by the owners themselves, not affiliated with this document.

Copyright © 2022 by Scott J. Barnard
All rights reserved. No part of this book may be reproduced, scanned, or distributed in any printed or electronic form without permission.

First Edition: March 2022

Cover: Illustration made by Diego Gilmar Valenzuela Astudillo

Printed in the United States of America

SCOTT J. BARNARD

THE METABOLIC
APPROACH TO OBESITY
4.0

Ultimate complete guide

Unlocking the Secrets of Weight Loss
Integrating Deep Nutrition, the Ketogenic Diet
and Nontoxic Bio-Individualized Therapies
and Intermittent Fasting for Women and Men

Scott J. Barnard

TABLE OF CONTENTS

CHAPTER 5 -

CHAPTER 6 -

CHAPTER 7 -

AUTHOR BIO -

Dedicated to all my friends and to all the people
who gave me their help.
Thanks a lot
Thanks to all of you for your confidence
in my qualities and what I do.
Scott J. Barnard

INTRODUCTION

The art of medicine is quite peculiar. Once in a while, medical treatments become established that don't really work. Through sheer inertia, these treatments get handed down from one generation of doctors to the next and survive for a surprisingly long time, despite their lack of effectiveness. Consider the medicinal use of leeches (bleeding) or, say, routine tonsillectomy. Unfortunately, the treatment of obesity is also one such example. Obesity is defined in terms of a person's body mass index, calculated as a person's weight in kilograms divided by the square of their height in meters. A body mass index greater than 30 is defined as obese. For more than thirty years, doctors have recommended a low-fat, calorie-reduced diet as the treatment of choice for obesity. Yet the obesity epidemic accelerates. Virtually every person who has used caloric reduction for weight loss has failed. And, really, who hasn't tried it? By every objective measure, this treatment is completely and utterly ineffective. Yet it remains the treatment of choice, defended vigorously by nutritional authorities.

Everybody, health professionals and patients alike, understood that the root cause of type 2 diabetes lay in weight gain. There were rare cases of highly motivated patients who had lost significant amounts of weight. Their type 2 diabetes would also reverse course. Logically, since weight was the underlying problem, it deserved significant attention. Still, it seemed that the health profession was not even the least bit interested in treating it. I was guilty as charged. Despite having worked for more than twenty years in medicine, I found that my own nutritional knowledge was rudimentary, at best. Treatment of this terrible disease— obesity—was left to large corporations like Weight Watchers, as well as various hucksters and charlatans mostly interested in peddling the latest weightloss "miracle." Doctors were not even remotely interested in nutrition. Instead, the medical profession seemed obsessed with finding and prescribing the next new drug:

- You have type 2 diabetes? Here, let me give you a pill.
- You have high blood pressure? Here, let me give you a pill.
- You have high cholesterol? Here, let me give you a pill.
- You have kidney disease? Here, let me give you a pill.

But all along, we needed to treat obesity. We were trying to treat the problems caused by obesity rather than obesity itself.

For example, Dr. Dean Ornish says that dietary fat is bad and carbohydrates are good. He is a respected doctor, so we should listen to him. But Dr. Robert Atkins said dietary fat is good and carbohydrates are bad. He was also a respected doctor, so we should listen to him. Who is right? Who is wrong? In the science of nutrition, there is rarely any consensus about anything:

- Dietary fat is bad. No, dietary fat is good. There are good fats and bad fats.

- Carbohydrates are bad. No, carbohydrates are good. There are good carbs and bad carbs.

You should eat more meals a day. No, you should eat fewer meals a day. Count your calories. No, calories don't count.

- Milk is good for you. No, milk is bad for you.
- Meat is good for you. No, meat is bad for you.

To discover the answers, we need to turn to evidence-based medicine rather than vague opinion. Literally thousands of books are devoted to dieting and weight loss, usually written by doctors, nutritionists, personal trainers and other "health experts." However, with a few exceptions, rarely is more than a cursory thought spared for the actual causes of obesity. What makes us gain weight? Why do we get fat?

The major problem is the complete lack of a theoretical framework for understanding obesity. Current theories are ridiculously simplistic, often taking only one factor into account:

- Excess calories cause obesity.
- Excess carbohydrates cause obesity.
- Excess meat consumption causes obesity.
- Excess dietary fat causes obesity.
- Too little exercise causes obesity

But all chronic diseases are multifactorial, and these factors are not mutually exclusive. They may all contribute to varying degrees. For example, heart disease has numerous contributing factors—family history, gender, smoking, diabetes, high cholesterol, high blood pressure and a lack of physical activity, to name only a few—and that fact is well accepted. But such is not the case in obesity research. The other major barrier to understanding is the focus on short-term studies. Obesity usually takes decades to fully develop. Yet we often rely on information about it from studies that are only of several weeks' duration. If we study how rust develops, we would need to observe metal over a period of weeks to months, not hours. Obesity, similarly, is a long-term disease. Short-term studies may not be informative.

While I understand that the research is not always conclusive, I hope this book, which draws on what I've learned over twenty years of helping patients with obesity lose weight permanently to manage their disease, will provide a structure to build upon. The process of challenging current nutritional dogma is, at times, unsettling, but the health consequences are too important to ignore. What actually causes weight gain and what can we do about it? This question is the overall theme of this book. A fresh framework for the understanding and treatment of obesity represents a new hope for a healthier future.

Some of you may have picked up this book to shed a few pounds for a special occasion, while others may have a more significant amount of weight to lose. Some of you have found that taking weight off is relatively easy but keeping it off long term is a lifelong challenge. Maybe you have simply been single too long and want to make a concerted attempt to look more attractive to the opposite sex. Maybe you're a parent trying to help your overweight child gain control of his or her eating habits. There is no bad reason to begin on this journey to lose weight, heal your body, and regain a second youth.

After you complete the 10-Day Green Smoothie Cleanse, you should transition to the DHEMM System, a permanent weight-loss system that will help you reach your desired weight. THE DHEMM System stands for:

- DETOX: Use one of the many detox methods described in this book
- HORMONAL BALANCE: Optimize your hormones for weight loss
- EAT CLEAN: Eat healthy, whole, and unprocessed foods
- MENTAL MASTERY: Achieve the right mental focus to stay motivated
- MOVE: Get moving and increase your physical activity

The DHEMM System is a breakthrough permanent weight-loss solution that melts fat from your body, especially from stubborn areas like the hips, thighs, and belly, through detoxifying and cleansing the body and feeding it healthy, nutrient-rich foods that keep it slim. Even if obesity runs in your family, you can break that hereditary cycle with this new approach to managing your weight. You can't change your genes, but by simply eating smart, you can manage how your body functions to optimize your health. I suggest you read this book just for understanding at first and then reread it with a mind to take action and begin your journey. Get a copy for a family member and friend so that you all can encourage and support one another through this life-changing transformation. Your family, friends, and I will be here to guide you along and support you. I have had frustrations with unexplained weight gain. I have worked hard to lose weight, only to find that each week, the pounds continued to pile on. You are not alone. We will do this together. Let your journey begin today.

Scott J. Barnard

CHAPTER 1

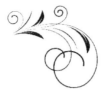

WHAT MAKES US OVERWEIGHT AND UNHEALTHY

I believe that most overweight people are actually naturally thin. The body is complex and designed to maintain healthiness. The body is smarter than any diet pill or fad diet on the market. If you just change your eating habits to align with your body's natural ability to heal, stay slim, and have energy, you will never have to worry about weight again. So, in this book, we are going to change the way you think about weight loss and eating forever. People who do not struggle with weight problems seem to think the cause of obesity is simply laziness and gluttony. In fact, I really get tired of people assuming that overweight or obese people should just eat less and exercise more to lose weight. This is an overly simplistic view of the problem. The mantra of "eat less and exercise more" does not solve the many complicated factors affecting weight gain for most people. You need to understand that the human body is much more complex than this as it relates to weight loss.

I've heard everything from "stop eating so much" and "step away from the table" to "overweight people are lazy and have no willpower." It's a false message to send to overweight people that being fat is totally their fault. This is simply not true. We may have heard an overweight person say, "I don't really eat that much, and I still can't seem to lose weight." Often they are telling the truth. In fact, I think we all know people who are overweight who work very hard to lose weight to no avail. They count calories, eat less, and work out but get little in the way of long-term or permanent results.

The truth is that nobody wants to be fat. Excess weight is due to a combination of factors that are often outside of one's control, such as genetics, hormonal imbalances, or the poor-quality Standard American Diet (SAD) readily available to us. It isn't your fault that you have problems with your weight. Even if you have enough willpower to keep yourself from eating when your brain tells you that you're hungry, you still may not be able to lose weight. There are so many other factors in play that cause you to gain weight. Until you understand the real reasons you gain weight, you will never be able to lose weight permanently. The key is to learn to naturally speed up your body's fat-burning capabilities to help you lose weight and get healthy.

There is no one simple reason why an individual may have trouble with his or her weight; in most cases, there are several reasons. I will share all of them with you so you can understand how to assist your own body in becoming naturally thin and healthy.

Why Diets Fail You

Diets are not the most effective way to lose weight permanently. Your goal should be to change your lifestyle, including proper nutrition and getting physically active, as a way to achieve your weight-loss goals. When most people think of dieting, they immediately think of eating less, which is a flawed dieting technique that allows you to lose weight in the short term but rarely allows you to keep the weight off permanently.

Even if you achieve your weight-loss goals through a particular diet, you will slowly gain the weight right back. The problem is that you "go on" a diet, which implies that you also later "go off" the diet. A typical diet is something you do for a short period of time. Therein lies the reason 95 percent of people who lose weight on a diet gain it back. In fact, if someone tells me they've lost twenty or thirty pounds on some great new diet, I tell them to come back in six months' time. If they have maintained their weight loss, then I'm willing to listen about this great new diet. By then, in many cases, they have unfortunately already begun to gain all the weight back.

Too many diets force you to eat bland, prepackaged, unappetizing food or chalky-tasting milkshakes. This causes you to crave and fantasize about all the delicious foods you can't have on your diet. These cravings or mental images challenge your willpower and cause you to give in to the foods you're missing, making you feel like you've failed on your diet again. My plan allows you to discover whole, natural foods that are healthy and palatable, without the empty calories. The beauty of fresh, whole foods is that you can eat them abundantly and still lose weight. When you eat high-sugar/high-fat foods, you tend to keep on eating and eating because sugar and fat don't make us feel full and cause us to crave more sugar and fat. However, whole, natural foods (fruits, veggies, whole grains) are nutrient-rich, high in fiber, and make us feel full and satisfied so we don't overeat.

Diets require that you eat less and lower your calorie intake, but if you don't provide your body with adequate nutrition, it will go into starvation mode and begin to hold on to fat for future use. Fat cells respond to starvation by holding on to the fat they already have as a survival mechanism, making it more difficult to shed fat in the long run. However, if you give your body the proper nutrition, it will shed fat, and the pounds will melt away without you even making an effort. When we consistently provide the body with good nutrition, the brain no longer believes the body is dieting, so it "relaxes" and stops telling the body to hold on to fat. As an example, if you skip breakfast to cut calories and lose weight, your stomach will begin to growl and send a message to your brain that you are starving, and it will immediately begin to store fat for future use in case your body does not receive any more food.

Any diet that deprives us of nutrients works against our weight-loss efforts. Even if you decide to lower your caloric intake, you still must be sure to eat high-quality foods that contain a lot of nutrients and vitamins. This is the key to losing weight.

Why Calorie Counting Is Useless

Most diets focus on restricting calories partly by cutting back on the amount of food eaten. But calorie restriction doesn't work in and of itself; losing weight is not just about eating less. In fact, if you eat too little, you set off a chain of chemical imbalances in your hormones and brain that actually cause you to gain weight. Yes, calories are important. But it is not the number of calories you consume as much as it is the type of calories that makes all the difference in how much weight you lose and how healthy you are. You can actually have an identical amount of calories from sugary foods (cupcake) and lean proteins (turkey breast), but the metabolic effect will be entirely different. The nutrients in sugary foods are different from the nutrients in lean proteins, and so they cause a different hormonal response, which plays a key role in determining what happens to those calories, such as how much of them end up being stored as fat in the body. This is why calorie counting simply does not work for weight loss.

What is a calorie? A calorie is simply a unit of energy. A more scientific definition states it as the quantity of energy required to raise the temperature of one gram of water by one degree Celsius under standard conditions. Simply stated, calories are units of energy that fuel our bodies, just as gasoline fuels our cars. We get calories from the food we eat. When we consume food, our body breaks down this food and turns it into energy. We consume calories so that we will have something to burn. The average adult body needs at least 1,000 to 1,400 calories to have enough energy to fuel key organs like the heart, brain, and lungs—to keep the basic functions of our body operating. This minimum number of calories is called your resting metabolic rate (RMR) and it varies depending upon your sex, age, weight, and muscle mass. You then need some additional calories (400 to 600) just to move and be active throughout the day. When you severely restrict caloric intake, it causes the number of calories you consume to drop below your resting metabolic rate. This then falls below the basic amount of energy or calories you need to fuel your body for the day.

The commonly stated logic is that if you eat the same number of calories you burn, you will stay the same weight. If you eat less than you burn, you will lose weight; if you eat more calories than you burn, you will gain weight. This seems to make sense, but it does not tell the whole story. As an example, let's look at the difference between 1,000 calories of lima beans versus 1,000 calories of a low-fat cinnamon raisin bagel. As far as calories go, they are both 1,000 calories. But because each item has a different amount of protein, fat, carbs, and fiber, the nutrients are absorbed into the body at different rates, sending different metabolic signals that ultimately control your weight. The carbs (sugar) from the lima beans enter your bloodstream very slowly, but the carbs from the low-fat cinnamon raisin bagel enter your bloodstream very rapidly. The calories from the lima beans will be absorbed over time and thus used over a longer period of time for energy. However, the calories from the cinnamon raisin bagel go into your bloodstream all at once, and any calories that can't be used right away for energy will get stored as fat. This mean the low-fat cinnamon raisin bagel causes more fat storage in the body, even though it has the same number of calories as the lima beans. Here's the general rule of thumb: foods whose calories enter your bloodstream quickly promote weight gain, whereas foods whose calories enter your bloodstream slowly promote weight loss. So, you can see why calorie counting alone is not effective for managing weight loss.

We are not going to be counting calories in the DHEMM System. I never count calories. For generations, people stayed slim and healthy without ever counting calories. Decades ago, people weren't focused on counting calories to stay slim, and obesity wasn't a widespread issue like it is today. Part of that reason is that they didn't eat all the processed foods and low-fat, low-calorie "diet" foods that we do today. So many people have messed up their metabolism by focusing on reducing calories that they ended up not getting the proper nutrition they needed to feed their body to stay slim and healthy. You can lose weight on 2,000 calories per day of clean, nutrient-rich foods and gain weight on 1,500 calories per day of junk food. If you are used to counting calories and have had success with that method to help control your weight, then by all means continue counting calories. However, if you do not have success with counting calories, you'll want to focus on what you're eating, the type of foods you're eating, and how they affect your weight loss.

The Importance of Detoxifying to Lose Weight

Another reason traditional diets so often don't work is that they don't address the toxic waste in the body. Simply counting calories does not detoxify and cleanse the body. Weight loss won't be permanent if your body's systems are sluggish or impacted with waste matter or you suffer from toxic overload. In the DHEMM System, we ensure that you first rid your body of toxins, sludge, and excess waste to ensure that it can best utilize and metabolize the food you eat. It is imperative that you detoxify the body to break the addiction to the foods that make you overweight and unhealthy in order to lose weight and keep it off. The method of dieting that involves resisting foods for a period of time and then returning to old eating habits will always cause the weight to return. Therefore, the goal is to break the addiction to foods that cause you to be overweight so you no longer desire or crave them anymore. Most traditional diets don't address how detoxifying the body aids in permanent weight loss.

Why Popular Diets Fail Us

There are many people who have tried popular diets but still struggle to lose the weight permanently. The primary reason is that most of the popular diets lack the nutritional support to allow your body to naturally regulate and lose weight. The diets often work in the short term, but they can also cause health problems, such as bloating, constipation, fatigue, skin problems, or make current health conditions worse due to the lack of balanced nutrition. Additionally, these diets don't address the underlying hormonal imbalances and sluggish metabolism issues that cause weight gain. Let's look at some of the current and popular diets and why they don't work for permanent weight loss.

High-protein/low-carb diets: Some of the most popular diets of our generation involve reducing or eliminating the intake of carbohydrates. When you do this, you will lose weight, but eliminating an entire food group removes nutrients the body needs to function properly. On this type of diet, you can eat large amounts of protein and fat and still continue to lose weight. The main problem with high-protein/low-carb diets is that they severely restrict an entire food group that has essential nutrients. Carbohydrates, such as grains, fruits, and vegetables, are what give us energy. When you stop eating carbohydrates, your body begins to break down fat very rapidly to receive a substitute for the carbohydrates it is no longer getting. This causes fat loss, initially. But your body will burn only a small amount of fat before it stops using fat as an energy source. It then begins to burn off water and then muscle tissue. In more serious cases, it will turn to connective tissue and then organ tissue. This process is called catabolism, and it can become extremely dangerous, even deadly. Eventually, melatonin and serotonin are not produced, which suppresses your ability to function normally and maintain energy. High-protein/low-carb diets can cause low energy, fatigue, sleeplessness, mental confusion, fainting, and vomiting. You will lose weight, but unfortunately, you will gain it back when you go off the diet.

Low-fat diets: Low-fat diets are among the most unsuccessful of all diets. Too many people focus on reducing and limiting all fat in their diet. We now know that healthy fats are a vital part of the body's survival and balance. The body's use of fat helps determine the satisfaction level a person receives from food. It helps to produce key hormones that assist with proper functioning of the brain. When low-fat diets became popular, many companies began offering low-fat versions of their products. But if you read the labels, many of these low-fat foods actually contain more calories than the regular version. This is due to the sugar added to make up for the flavor that was lost when fat was eliminated from the product. If you eat these foods, you really aren't making much progress toward your weight-loss goals while on a low-fat diet. So many people end up eating low-fat foods and snacks thinking they were working toward losing weight, when in actuality they were eating more sugar and calories than they had in the past.

High-carbohydrate diets: A high-carb diet has a lot of potatoes, breads, pastas, grains, and rice—so-called "energy" foods. Although carbs are necessary for a well-balanced diet, too many carbs can have a negative effect on blood-sugar levels, which affects mood and brain functioning. Additionally, too many carbs can create a condition known as insulin resistance, which I'll discuss later. Insulin resistance is a common, but not widely known, reason so many people are getting fat at an alarming rate. Additionally, carbs tend to have more calories than other foods. In the long term, a high-carb diet prevents the body from burning fat for fuel. So even though you may initially lose weight, you will quickly gain more weight, namely fat.

As I have often said, it's not hard to lose weight rapidly, but the trick is to keep the weight off permanently. Permanent weight loss must come from burning fat and maintaining as much lean muscle mass as possible. You want to eliminate toxic overload in the body to shrink your fat cells. You want to also be sure that your hormones are properly balanced and that they are not hindering your weight-loss goals. Permanent weight loss (or fat loss) can be achieved with knowledge and effort as long as you remember that people don't fail at diets; diets fail people. Most diets simply don't help you achieve permanent weight loss.

Why Exercise Won't Make You Thin

Is exercising good for your health? Sure! Is it key to losing weight? Absolutely not! But so many people believe that it is. We've all heard the mantra "eat less and exercise more to lose weight." Close to 50 million Americans have gym memberships or belong to health clubs. We spend about $20 billion a year on gym memberships, yet obesity rates continue to drastically increase year after year. There are many good reasons to exercise, such as improving cardiovascular health, but weight loss is not one of them. The truth of the matter is that although exercise is important for good health, the foods you eat are three times more important for controlling your weight than exercise. I remember reading a Time magazine cover story that quoted the prominent exercise researcher and professor Eric Ravussin, who admitted to Time ("Why Exercise Won't Make You Thin," August 9, 2009) that "in general, for weight loss, exercise is pretty useless."

To lose one pound of fat by exercising, you must burn 3,500 calories. This would be equivalent to running thirty-five miles or walking on a treadmill for about seven and a half hours (at four miles per hour). As you can see, it would take a considerable amount of exercise to make a huge impact on your weight-loss goals. I think it is important to note that exercise has many more benefits beyond weight loss. Most people who take up exercise become healthier by increasing their aerobic activity, which results in decreased blood pressure and overall better mood and mental health. I think because exercise is good for your overall health, many health practitioners downplay the fact that more and more research has shown that exercise has a negligible impact on weight loss. In other words, exercise may not be critical for weight loss, but in general, it is still great for our overall health.

It is true that exercise burns calories, and you must burn calories to lose weight, but exercise has another effect that counteracts the burning of calories: it stimulates hunger, which causes you to eat more, which in turn offsets any weight lost from exercising. Exercise doesn't necessarily make you lose weight; in fact, it could make you gain some. The one time in my life that I worked out with a trainer for a few months, I gained fifteen pounds. When I complained to my trainer, he said the extra weight was all muscle. But my feeling was Who cares? I can't fit into my clothes. And I hated my new body shape—not curvy and shapely, but big and bulky. Even though I feel it is one of my personal flaws, I have to be honest with you: I don't work out. I haven't exercised in years. I tried to in the past but could never stick with it for more than four months, even when I had a trainer. I know that it's good for me and that we should all exercise, but unfortunately, I don't have the discipline to stick to an exercise regimen.

However, I do have a strong desire to look and feel great. So I had to figure out how I could lose weight and keep it off, knowing that I didn't want to do fad diets and didn't want to be in the gym all the time. Happily, I found a system of healthy living that has yielded amazing results: permanent weight loss, a higher energy level, and overall great health! As a result, I have come to the conclusion that staying slim is all about eating right, while being fit is about exercising. So, as long as I focus on healthy eating, I will continue to stay slim. But if I want to reach a high level of fitness, I will need to incorporate more exercise into my life.

The question we should be asking ourselves is how much physical activity we need to be healthy and fit. Physical activity is about movement—things that get you moving throughout the day and away from the computer, TV, bed, or couch. Exercise is a type of physical activity where you set aside a specified amount of time to get moving. You can be physically active throughout the course of the day without ever going to the gym. People tend to greatly overestimate how many calories they burn while "exercising." The reality is that walking on a treadmill for about an hour burns only 350 to 400 calories, which can be nullified with one jelly donut or one or two glasses of wine. People typically burn 200 to 300 calories in a 30- minute aerobic-exercise session, but when they follow it up with a bottle of Gatorade, they replace all the calories they just burned. Another way to think of it is that you have to do a lot more exercise than the average person does in a typical hour-long session to burn off about 500 calories. To burn off just two donuts, about 500 calories, takes roughly two hours of cycling.

To burn off two slices of pepperoni pizza, you'd have to do one and a half hours of swimming. So you have to do an awful lot more exercise than most people realize to make any real progress toward weight loss. For some time, researchers have been finding that people who exercise don't necessarily lose weight. An increasing body of work reveals that exercise is rather ineffective when it comes to losing weight unless eating habits are also changed. Changing how and what you eat is the most effective route for losing weight. So, practically speaking, exercise is not the most effective method for slimming down unless you have the training regimen of an Olympian or professional athlete. I definitely don't want to give people an excuse to not exercise; rather, I want them to accurately understand what exercise can and cannot do for their weight-loss goals. Those of you who do exercise should be proud of yourselves, and I encourage you to keep it up. When you get more physically active, you feel better about yourself and feel more inclined to watch the type of foods you put in your body.

In a very noteworthy experiment led by Dr. Timothy Church at the Louisiana State University, who published his results in the prestigious Journal of the American Medical Association, hundreds of overweight women were put on exercise regimens for a six-month period for the purpose of determining the health benefits of exercise. One group worked out for 70 minutes each week, another for 135 minutes, another for 190 minutes, and another kept to their normal daily routine with no additional exercise. The women in the study were all postmenopausal, sedentary, overweight, and had elevated blood pressure. To ensure there was 100 percent compliance with the exercise regimens, the women's exercising was supervised to accurately monitor results.

It was found that there was no significant difference in weight loss between those who had exercised, even with some groups exercising for several hours per week, and those who did not exercise. In fact, some of the women who exercised even gained weight. The possible reason for this was a problem identified as "compensation." Those who did exercise canceled out the calories they had just burned by eating more, typically as a self-reward (rewarding yourself with food) for working out or to satisfy their stimulated appetites from the actual workout. It would be as if I would eat a donut or pastry to celebrate all the hard effort that I just put in during my workout, but in reality, I simply erased all the calories that were burned. So if you have committed to exercising, and that is indeed a good thing, be sure not to get in the habit of rewarding yourself with food.

One positive finding in the study was that every exercise group reported an improvement in quality of life, including the group that exercised for ten minutes a day. That means that as little as ten minutes of exercise a day has benefits. This is very good news for those who can find only ten to fifteen minutes a day for exercise but are not able to find one hour three times a week. Barry Braun, associate professor of kinesiology at the University of Massachusetts, found that the evidence emerging from his research team shows that moderate exercise, such as "low-intensity ambulation" (i.e., walking), may help to burn calories "without triggering a caloric compensation effect," meaning you won't immediately feel the need for a snack after your workout as a result of increased appetite hormones in your blood. This means that an intense workout in the gym might actually be less effective than gentle exercises, such as walking, in terms of weight loss because you don't get the stimulated appetite that comes with intense workouts.

If you look at numerous studies over the years, it clearly shows exercise alone won't make you thin; rather, being physically active is a key factor in weight loss. In the DHEMM System, we focus on ways to get physically active throughout the day as opposed to just exercising a few times a week. Even if you just do light exercise—like taking a brisk walk to and from lunch or walking up the stairs instead of taking the elevator—you will get many of the good benefits of exercise. This is because light exercise can increase your heart rate and improve your cardiovascular health. Another consideration is that once you become overweight, it is much harder to exercise or go to the gym to work out. However, you are more likely to be able to simply "get moving" throughout the day. Once you begin to lose weight and become healthier, it will be easier to incorporate more intense physical activity (i.e., exercise) into your daily regimen.

I strongly believe that nutritional education must come first. People don't lack willpower; they lack nutritional education. Eating habits must change first with a focus on nutrient-rich foods that do not cause the body to gain and store fat. I believe that changing how and what you eat will help you lose weight. Being physically active helps you keep the weight off permanently, so you'll find two key steps of the DHEMM System are to EAT (healthy, nutrient-rich foods) and to MOVE (get physically active throughout the day). Since we know being physically active is good for your overall health, it makes sense to focus on that as well as changing your eating habits.

Why A Sugar Addiction Is Worse Than A Drug Addiction

Many people are addicted to sugar and don't even know it. I believe this addiction is the main reason people get fat. They don't think they eat a lot of sugar because they don't eat a lot of candy, cakes, and pies, but the problem is that sugar is hidden in many foods, including breads, muffins, and even dried fruit. I believe sugar is toxic. It has no nutritional value, it's highly addictive, and it makes you sick and fat. Certain types of foods, such as processed foods and simple carbohydrates (candy, sugar, sweets), are high in sugar, toxic to our digestive system, and cause us to gain weight and make poor food choices in the long run. Processed foods and simple carbohydrates (sugar) are low in nutrients and high in calories. Many of us have heard that excess sugar consumption can lead to food cravings, binge eating, and, worst of all, sugar addiction. Sugar stimulates the dopamine and opioid receptors of the brain, which are the same receptors stimulated by other addictive substances, such as cocaine and morphine. Just like those drugs, sugar can become addictive. If you try to cut back or break your addiction to sugar, you will experience withdrawal symptoms, the same as a drug addict does. Over time, having an excess of refined sugar in the diet leads to not only weight gain but also other serious diseases, like heart disease, stroke, or type 2 diabetes.

Dr. Judith J. Wurtman, a nutritionist at MIT, has shown that eating refined carbohydrates like cookies, cakes, candy, pasta, or white bread raises serotonin and endorphins in the brain, creating a happy, feel-good, peaceful state. This is why we crave these carbs when we're anxious or stressed. However, you only "feel good" in the short term and then you crave more in order to remain in that happy state. You begin self-medicating with food— eating sweets to make yourself feel balanced and calm. No matter if you crave sweets or breads or pasta, it all has the same effect because it all converts quickly to sugar in your body and causes you to crave more of the same.

How Sugar Makes You Fat

When you eat sugar, it gets stored in the liver in the form of glycogen. When the liver is overloaded with sugar, it begins to expand, and when it is maxed out, the glycogen is expelled in the form of fatty acids. This excess fat —called fatty acid— is deposited into areas such as the belly, butt, thighs, and hips. Where it gets most dangerous is when the remaining fatty acids end up in our major organs, including the heart and kidneys. Sugary foods (candy, cakes, pies, muffins, and sodas) and other refined, starchy carbohydrates cause a rapid rise in insulin levels, which results in excess fat in the body. When food is eaten, it is broken down to glucose so it can be used to fuel the body. Insulin is the hormone that sends glucose out of the blood into the tissue cells for use as energy. When excess glucose remains in the blood, insulin levels stay high. Chronically elevated insulin can cause both fat storage and more inflammation in the body. When insulin levels are high, this is a signal to the body to store extra calories as fat and to refrain from burning fat. High insulin levels mean you'll have more body fat, while low insulin levels mean you'll have less body fat.

Research has also shown that a high-sugar diet causes cancer cells to multiply rapidly. An important study published in the medical journal Cancer Research was conducted by a team out of the University of California, Los Angeles. The researchers found that while sugar of any kind offered sustenance to cancer cells, fructose played a key role in the proliferation of cancer cells. That means that cancer spreads more quickly on a high-fructose diet. The food industry has been extremely successful at designing foods to capture the hearts and minds of those who enjoy food. Food manufacturers and restaurant owners may not fully understand the science behind why sugar, salt, and fat sell so well, but they know that they do. Thus, they make foods that are laden with sugar, salt, and fat. When food appeals to our taste buds, we say that it is palatable. But scientists know that food that is palatable stimulates our appetite and cravings and causes us to eat more of it.

In fact, we become motivated to pursue that taste over and over again. Eating foods high in sugar and salt makes us want to eat more foods that are high in sugar and salt. Eating foods that taste good causes us to eat more food that tastes good. The average American's sugar load is about a hundred pounds per year. We have become physically addicted to simple carbohydrates (candy, sugar, sweets). In a 2007 study conducted in France, cocaine-addicted rats were offered super-sweetened water using a combination of sugar and artificial sweeteners. In just three days, the cocaine-addicted rats switched their allegiance from cocaine to the super-sweetened sugar water. The conclusion was that sugar activates dopamine receptors just as cocaine does. But unlike cocaine, sugar has no adverse effects on the nervous system. When the rats got a hit of sugar, they gained the highs of cocaine without the downside of increased nervousness. Since cocaine is known to be one of the most addictive substances on earth, we can see how humans can so easily get addicted to sugar. Sugar gives them the same effect of the hit on their dopamine receptors as cocaine does. Humans can easily become addicted to sugar and go through withdrawal if they can't get sugar quickly.

Are You Addicted to Sugar?

If you answer yes to more than ten of these questions, then chances are that you are a sugar addict.

- Do you put sugar in coffee or tea?
- Do you drink sodas at least once a day?
- Do you drink sweetened fruit punches, sports drinks, or juices?
- Do you use syrups, jams, or jellies several times a week?
- Did you eat a lot of candy growing up as a kid?
- Do you crave sweets, pasta, or breads or are they your favorite foods?
- Do you eat bread, bagels, croissants, muffins, or donuts for breakfast?
- Do you feel chronically tired or fatigued most days?
- Do you often eat a dessert after dinner?
- Do you crave sweets in the afternoon or late at night?
- Do you buy candy at the movie theater?

- Do you have headaches often?
- Do you drink fruity or sweetened alcoholic drinks?
- Do you keep candy or snacks in your home at all times?
- Do you eat sweets first at a happy hour or party?

How to Break the Sugar Addiction

Are you having a panic attack right now just thinking about giving up sugar? You have to look at kicking the sugar habit as though you are ending an addiction. The key is to understand where your sugar is coming from and then find alternatives to eating so much sugar in your foods. Start by making yourself aware of everything that has sugar in it. First, you must know how to find sugar in your foods, as it is cleverly hidden in the labeling. Virtually everything we eat, especially packaged and processed foods—including diet and low-fat foods—has sugar in it. You will want to read labels to determine the total amount of sugar in the products you buy and to check the list of ingredients for the names of things that are really just sugar in disguise. Refined white sugar, or table sugar, which is sucrose, is the form of sugar that is most familiar to people.

However, the other sugars that are commonly found in food are listed on labels as high fructose corn syrup, glucose, fructose (fruit sugar), dextrose (corn sugar), maltose (malt sugar), lactose (milk sugar), corn sweetener, raw sugar, brown sugar, powdered sugar, molasses, and maple sugar. Begin by looking at your drinks and the packaged goods in your refrigerator and pantry. Get rid of those foods that have a high sugar content (5 grams of sugar or more per serving). Sugar is measured in grams, and 4 grams of sugar equals one teaspoon. So if your soda has 40 grams of sugar, that's about ten teaspoons of sugar in just one soda. You can see how so many people end up eating so much sugar every day. I used to think I was consuming a healthy breakfast by eating oatmeal. However, it wasn't regular oatmeal but the sweetened, flavored instant oatmeal, like apple-cinnamon oatmeal, and it had about 20 grams of sugar per serving, which is way too much.

Remember, as a guideline, the best way to minimize the amount of sugar in your diet is to choose foods that have 5 grams or less per serving. When the drink or food item has 5 grams or less of sugar per serving size, the body doesn't overreact to the sugar. This means your pancreas will not have to release too much insulin, which can cause fat storage in the body. (I'll explain this concept in a later section.) To sweeten foods, it is always better to use stevia or some equivalent herbal sweetener rather than sugar. Stevia is a natural sweetener made from a plant native to South America. Other countries have been using stevia as a sugar substitute for several decades since it is virtually calorie-free and does not affect blood glucose, which makes it a great natural alternative to sugar and artificial sweeteners.

When you crave sweets, try fruit as a better alternative. In fact, it is your best defense against insulin spikes and cravings. Facing these cravings is the beginning of detoxifying and rebalancing your body. The cravings will actually disappear after three to four days. And once you fight these cravings, your cravings won't be as strong as long as you continue to keep high-sugar foods out of your diet. Sugar will cause you to get fat; feel irritable, moody, and tired; and can cause all kinds of health problems, so commit to breaking your sugar addiction today.

How Toxins Make You Fat, Sick, And Tired

I was coaching a client when she asked me a very poignant question: "why am I always sick, and what's making me fat?" I said, "That is not the question of the day, but the question of the century." Toxins make us fat and sick! And they are the missing piece to the puzzle as to why we can't lose weight and why we feel unhealthy and tired!

What Are Toxins?

A toxin is any substance that irritates or creates harmful effects in the body or mind. Toxins are everywhere, and we are unknowingly filling our bodies with them every day. There are two types of toxins: environmental toxins and internal toxins.

• Environmental toxins are found outside the body/mind and include pollutants, smog, medications, hormones/birth control pills, household cleaners, food additives, and pesticides.

• Internal toxins are found inside the body/mind and include bacterial/yeast/fungal overgrowth, parasite infections, chronic worry or fear, food allergies, and dental or medical implants, such as implants from cosmetic surgeries, joint replacements, or mercury dental fillings. We live in a sea of toxins. You cannot avoid them, but you can help your body get rid of some of them. Every person on the planet has residues of toxic chemicals or metals in their tissues. Some 80,000 new chemicals have been introduced since the turn of the twentieth century, and most have never been tested for safety or for how they interact in the human body. Our air is toxic; our water is polluted; our food is depleted of nutrients and packed with poisonous chemicals and hormones. Not only that, but our minds and hearts often get polluted also.

Toxins create a heavy burden in the body, which causes many of the body's systems to malfunction. The buildup of toxins overwhelms the body's vital organs and other systems, creating an array of health issues, including fatigue, memory loss, premature aging, skin eruptions/acne, depression, arthritis, hormone imbalances, chronic fatigue, anxiety, emotional disorders, muscle and joint pain, cancers, heart disease, and much, much more. There's no delicate way of putting this, but to some extent, we're all toxic, which is one of the biggest reasons so many people are overweight. Just because you are overweight does not guarantee that you have a toxic overload, and just because you are thin does not mean that you do not have a toxic overload. We have to evaluate our toxic overload individually, regardless of whether we are slim or fat. However, it is rare that an overweight person who rids the body of excess toxins does not lose weight.

Please know that getting rid of the fat by exercising or dieting doesn't necessarily get rid of the toxins. Toxins just get reabsorbed by your body, creating new fat cells, which makes losing weight without getting rid of the toxins a hinder to permanent weight loss. Some research data implies that the obesity epidemic in the United States is due to toxic overload. An article in the April 2002 issue of The Journal of Alternative and Complementary Medicine concluded the following: "The commonly held causes of obesity such as overeating and inactivity do not explain the current obesity epidemic. Because the obesity epidemic occurred rather quickly, it has been suggested that environmental causes instead of genetic factors may be largely responsible." In other words, they are suggesting that the environmental chemicals (i.e., toxins) that have increased in number over the last one hundred years may help explain the widespread obesity epidemic.

Having monitored human exposure to toxic environmental chemicals since 1972, the Environmental Protection Agency (EPA) began the National Human Adipose Tissue Survey to evaluate the levels of various toxins in fat tissue. The study found that five of what are known to be the most toxic chemicals (OCDD or octachlorodibenzo-p-dioxin, styrene, dichlorobenzene, xylene, and ethylphenol) were found in 100 percent of all tissue samples. These toxic chemicals from industrial pollution damage the liver, heart, lungs, and nervous system. Additionally, nine more chemicals were found in 91 to 98 percent of samples, including benzene, toluene, ethylbenzene, and DDE. These toxins found in the fat tissues not only contribute to our weight issues but are also damaging our health. The good news is that one way to get rid of excess toxins in the body is by changing the thing that caused it in the first place, which is diet. In the DHEMM System, we provide foods that help you rid the body of toxins, resulting in improved energy, health, and vitality.

Toxic Overload in Your Body

Toxic overload refers to the level of toxins found in tissues of the human body by analysis of the blood and urine. Toxins are stored in almost every tissue in the body, including fat, skeletal muscle, bones, tendons, joints/ligaments, and visceral organs. When the body is properly nourished and detoxified, its organs operate at peak performance. However, whenever our elimination channels become clogged due to toxic overload and poor diet, we should follow a comprehensive detoxification program to improve its functioning. Detoxification may still be unfamiliar to many but is really quite natural and beneficial. Just as we regularly clean our homes, our cars, and the outside of our bodies, we should cleanse our inner body. First, to get a sense of what the toxic load is in your body, take the quiz below.

If you are dealing with fatigue, weight gain, chronic disease, inability to focus, or accelerated aging, you will want to take this quiz to determine if toxic overload in your body is the underlying cause. Take this quiz and score your results to gain a sense of how much toxic burden you're carrying in your body.

Read each question and give yourself one point for every yes answer.

- Do you crave sweets, bread, pasta, white rice, and/or potatoes?
- Do you eat processed foods (TV dinners, lunchmeat) or fast foods at least three times a week?

- Do you drink caffeinated beverages like coffee and tea more than twice daily?
- Do you drink diet sodas or use artificial sweeteners at least once a day?
- Do you sleep less than eight hours per day?
- Do you drink less than 64 ounces of good, clean water daily?
- Are you very sensitive to smoke, chemicals, or fumes in the environment?
- Have you taken or are you taking antibiotics, antidepressants, or other medications?
- Do you take or have you taken birth control pills or other estrogens, such as hormone replacement therapy?
- Do you have frequent yeast infections?
- Do you have "silver" dental fillings?
- Do you use commercial household cleaners, cosmetics, or deodorants?
- Do you eat non-organic vegetables, fruits, or meat?
- Have you ever smoked or been exposed to secondhand smoke?
- Are you overweight or do you have cellulite fat deposits?
- Does your occupation expose you to environmental toxins?
- Do you live in a major metropolitan area or near a big airport?
- Do you feel tired, fatigued, or sluggish throughout the day?
- Do you have difficulty concentrating or focusing?
- Do you suffer bloating, indigestion, or frequent gas after eating?
- Do you get more than two colds or the flu per year?
- Do you have reoccurring congestion, sinus issues, or postnasal drip?
- Do you sometimes notice bad breath, a coated tongue, or strong smelling urine?
- Do you have puffy eyes or dark circles under your eyes?
- Are you often sad or depressed?
- Do you often feel anxious, antsy, or stressed?
- Do you have acne, breakouts, rashes, or hives?
- Do you have less than one bowel movement per day and/or get constipated occasionally?
- Do you have insomnia or trouble getting restful sleep?
- Do you get blurred vision or itchy, burning eyes?

The higher your score, the greater the potential toxic burden you may be carrying and the more you may benefit from a detoxification and cleansing program. If you scored 20 or higher, you will significantly benefit from detoxifying your body, which could lead to weight loss and improved health and vitality. If you scored between 5 and 19, you may benefit from a detoxification program for improved health and vitality. If you scored below 5, you might actually be free of toxic overload in the body and living a very healthy, toxin-free life. Good for you!

Signs of toxic overload in the body include the following:

- Bloating and gas

- Constipation
- Indigestion
- Low energy/fatigue
- Brain fog/depression
- Weight gain
- Chronic pain
- Infections
- Allergies
- Headaches

Toxic overload can also be identified through different tests that help determine your individual body burden. There are facilities that offer specialty testing to measure toxicity levels.

One of the most commonly held myths today is that the body can detoxify itself and does not need any help. You may have heard that the body can eliminate toxins on its own. Our body does naturally try to eliminate toxins, but overexposure to any of them will slow down the body's detoxification systems. The reality is that you can assist the body in detoxifying and eliminating toxins that cause weight gain and harm your health. You can and should detoxify and cleanse the body if you want to live better and live longer. Yes, toxins are real, they do exist, and the good news is that there are many ways to eliminate them from the body. In this book, I will provide the most practical and effective techniques to detoxify and cleanse the body.

Many people struggle on a diet because of their strong cravings. Cravings are not only a matter of willpower. They can actually be eliminated by properly detoxing and cleansing the body to eliminate waste and toxins. As I gained weight in my thirties, I learned that although my metabolism was beginning to slow due to aging, that wasn't the real reason why I couldn't lose weight. I learned that my excess weight was not all fat; some of it was waste in my body—excess toxic waste caused by years of poor eating, leading to fluid retention and intestinal waste matter in my colon.

Many in the medical industry will tell you that you do not need to help your body cleanse and detoxify. Yet, there is more and more scientific research that shows industrial and environmental toxins to be a factor in many diseases, such as Parkinson's. Most of the advice that comes from the medical community around weight loss focuses on eating less and exercising more. But I never trust my health and wellness solely to the medical community and really feel that I don't need a license in order to understand my body and health. I have the ultimate respect for doctors, but in my opinion, they are trained to treat symptoms and may not be as experienced in understanding the role toxic overload plays on our health issues and ailments. This is true, particularly if a doctor received his medical degree decades ago.

However, as with any change to your diet or lifestyle, you should consult with your physician as you begin your journey toward healthy eating and living. In fact, you may even enlighten him and provide valuable information that he can utilize in his practice to help other patients. We are all here to help one another toward great health. One of my favorite quotes is the following: "Health is a state of complete physical, mental, and social wellbeing and not merely the absence of disease or infirmity".

How Our Standard American Diet (SAD) Contributes to Toxic Overload in the Body

An important link between weight gain and toxic overload in the body is the quality of the food we eat. Food is our energy source, and the more nutritional the food, the better the body will function. If we choose foods that are nutrient-rich, organic, and free of toxins, the body will receive and absorb the highest nutrient intake, allowing us to feel satisfied and full without empty calories, which cause us to eat more and more. Yet we are eating less and less of these healthy, nutrient-rich foods today. The Standard American Diet (SAD) consists of highly processed and refined foods, including frozen foods, fast foods, and prepared foods that are canned, boxed, and processed to create "instant" varieties that are the least healthy for you. Restaurants, especially fast-food chains, and supermarkets are filled with foods high in fat, sugar, cholesterol, sodium, artificial flavors, pesticides, hormones, and preservatives, all of which contribute to the toxic overload in the body.

Let's take a closer look at the Standard American Diet that so many of us eat. It typically includes lots of highly refined wheat products, such as white bread, crackers, bagels, pasta, and cereals, as well as other processed foods, such as potato chips and corn chips. Don't forget the fatty meats like steaks, burgers, hot dogs, ribs, bacon, and pork chops. Now, top it all off with a large amount of saturated fat, hydrogenated oil, and processed vegetable oils, such as salad dressing, most cooking oils, and mayonnaise. It's no wonder we have an epidemic of heart disease, cancer, diabetes, and arthritis as well as many other degenerative diseases. Now, for dessert, we eat baked goods, such as cakes, pies, cupcakes, cookies, fudge, and brownies—and don't forget the donuts and candy bars. In many ways, former generations were some of the healthiest people on the planet because many of these foods did not exist.

But today, our lifestyle has become much too stressed and fast-paced to take time to eat healthy foods. However, we are supposed to eat in order to "feed" our body the nutrients it needs to maintain vitality and health. It's not just how much you're eating that's causing you to gain weight, it is also what you're eating and what your body is being exposed to that causes a toxic overload in your body. Even though we are not technically starving like some people in other areas of the world, we are definitely malnourished. We eat a lot, but our nutritional deficiencies manifest themselves as "belly fat," "thunder thighs," "underarm bat wings," "beer bellies," and "cottage cheese behind." Do any of these sound familiar?

How Toxins Cause Excess Fat in the Body

There are many factors that contribute to weight gain, and one factor that is most overlooked by traditional diets is toxic overload. Simply put, people often have difficulty losing weight because their bodies are full of poisons. The more toxins you take in or are exposed to every day, the more toxins you store in fat cells in the body. Toxins stored in fat cells are difficult to get rid of through dieting alone. You must first detoxify the body. When the body is overloaded with toxins, the body transfers its energy away from burning calories and uses that energy to work harder to detoxify the body. In other words, the body does not have the energy to burn calories. However, when the body is efficiently detoxifying and getting rid of toxins, the energy can be used to burn fat. Thus, the DHEMM System starts with detoxification as the first step in helping you shed pounds.

I believe the most effective weight-loss programs should focus on both fat loss and detoxification. Detoxification, which is the process of removing toxins from the body, is critical to losing fat because many of the toxins the body holds on to are stored in fat cells. When you begin to lose weight (fat), toxins stored in fat cells are released into the bloodstream and need to be eliminated from the body so they don't cause illness. Therefore, weight loss that includes detoxification results in not only fat loss but also overall improved health and wellness.

Your body stores the majority of toxins in fat cells, and it's actually safer for toxins to be in your fat cells than in your bloodstream. The downside to this is that the more body fat you have, the more toxins you are also storing. And because your body knows that releasing toxins into your bloodstream is less desirable than having them stored safely in your fat cells, it holds on to the fat cells for dear life and doesn't want to let them go, making it difficult for you to lose fat. Thus, fat cells don't break down very easily and they literally weigh down the body and make it bigger. So, the first step in losing weight is detoxification. Without detoxification, millions of people worldwide lose the fight to lose weight permanently. The more toxins the body is storing, the more fat it is likely to accumulate and retain. It is not by accident that American obesity levels are rising right alongside the increase in environmental toxins.

How Toxins Hinder Weight Loss

A study published in Obesity Reviews concluded that during weight loss, certain toxins (e.g., pesticides) are released from fat tissue where they are typically stored. These toxins can pollute your body, slow metabolism, and make additional weight loss more challenging. Additional studies suggest toxins released during weight loss interfere with thyroid and mitochondrial function, which disrupts your metabolic rate and reduces your body's ability to burn fat and calories. A study by Catherine Pelletier, a researcher at Laval University, supports how environmental toxins can also negatively affect your thyroid, which is critical for proper metabolism regulation. So it becomes imperative to take steps to detoxify the body if you plan to lose weight and excess body fat. This will allow for safer toxin elimination and avoid the slowing of your metabolism. Toxins can interfere with your ability to lose weight by:

• Slowing down your metabolism: As toxins are being released from fat cells, they may cause the thyroid to slow down, negatively impacting metabolism. When the thyroid slows down, so does metabolism, which leads to weight gain and low energy.

• Decreasing your ability to burn fat: Toxins hinder the body's ability to burn fat by up to 20 percent. Toxins released during weight loss interfere with mitochondrial function, which reduces your body's ability to burn fat.

• Slowing down the time it takes for you to feel full: There are hormones that send signals that tell the brain we are full so that we stop eating. Toxic overload causes hormonal imbalances that stop these signals from working properly.

• Interfering with our appetite systems: Besides directly lowering thyroid hormone levels, metabolic rate, and fat burning, toxins can damage the mechanisms that control appetite. Toxins can interfere with all the delicate appetite-control systems that are regulated by hormones and neurotransmitters from the fat cells, the gut, and brain.

Weight loss can be a challenge on its own, but when we add the fact that toxins residing in fat cells also play a factor, it is that much harder. If you had been making good progress losing weight and all of a sudden reached a plateau and can't lose those last twenty pounds, you may want to determine if toxic overload in your body is hindering your weight-loss progress.

CHAPTER 2

THE FIVE KEYS TO PERMANENT WEIGHT LOSS

There are five commandments to follow to achieve permanent weight loss, and all of them are addressed in the DHEMM System to ensure that you lose weight and keep it off. The five commandments are as follows:

1. Detoxify your body, primarily the liver, which must be able to properly metabolize sugars and fats so you can eliminate stubborn fat in the body.
2. Correct your hormonal imbalances so that your brain and gut communicate with one another to drive your eating behavior and control your appetite.
3. Learn how to accelerate your metabolism (metabolic engine) to turn your body into a fat-burning machine.
4. Eat foods that make you thin.
5. Avoid foods that make you fat.

Understanding the reasons for these five commandments will help you succeed not only in maintaining your ideal weight but also in managing your long-term health and even reversing chronic ailments and diseases. The consequence of these changes will result in effortless weight loss and a new feeling of life and renewed energy. You will enjoy delicious, healthy, nutritionist-designed food choices that have many fat-burning and healing properties.

Following these commandments is critical to long-term, sustainable weight loss that doesn't depend on eating less but rather on eating more nutrient-rich foods that help your body stay slim and healthy. While weight loss experts have emphasized one or two of these elements, no one has integrated these five critical success factors into a complete program until now. Following the DHEMM System will ensure you permanent weight loss and good health for the rest of your life.

Get Rid Of Toxic Overload In The Body

As discussed in the previous section, the first key to weight loss involves getting rid of toxins in the body. If you try to lose weight without getting rid of the toxins, then you're guaranteed to gain the weight right back—even if you exercise to burn fat. To lose weight permanently, you must detoxify and cleanse the body to get rid of toxins we encounter every day so they don't reenter the body and create more and more fat cells.

What Does It Mean to Detoxify the Body?

Detoxification is a total-body cleansing process for all of the body's detoxification organs and systems. Detoxification is the process of cleansing and reducing the toxic overload that currently resides in your body. Because there are so many toxins in your cells, tissues, and organs, you detoxify to bring them out of hiding so they can be eliminated from the body. Many people falsely think of the word "cleanse" as a one-time fast or colon cleanse you do for a few days every few years. This is detoxification in a very narrow sense. Although the colon is one of the many detoxification channels for elimination, total body cleansing goes far beyond colon cleansing. It involves cleansing all of the detox organs, including the liver, kidneys, skin, etc. Just as you wouldn't wait a year to clean your house, you shouldn't wait a year to "cleanse" your inner body. Regular cleansing ensures that you are constantly eliminating toxins and getting rid of waste and sludge. If you wait too long to cleanse the body, toxins get deeper into the body, making you look and feel tired and old, eventually leading to disease and weight gain. The goal is not to be camped out near a toilet all day, but rather to incorporate detoxification methods that are gradual but steady to avoid disruptive side effects. Thus, we have to think of cleansing as a regular, ongoing activity we do to reach our optimum health and wellness.

Detoxing differs from dieting in that its primary goal is to cleanse the entire body. However, one of the natural outcomes of detoxing is that excess weight melts away. The idea is to simply help the body in its natural process of self-cleansing. We are continually eliminating excess toxins through our digestive, urinary, circulatory, respiratory, and lymphatic systems as well as our skin. Helping the body cleanse is not unnatural. Some call the act of toxins being released from the tissues and cells "detoxification" while flushing the waste out or eliminating toxins from the body is "cleansing." For our purposes, we will refer to the entire process as detoxification or cleansing. In this book, the words detoxification, detox, and cleansing may be used interchangeably.

The benefits of detoxifying the body include:

- Weight loss and the realization that you can enjoy a lighter style of eating
- Improved digestion; better elimination; less constipation, gas, bloating, and indigestion
- Fewer allergic or reactive responses to foods
- Less mucus and congestion and the clearing up of sniffles and coughs
- More energy, better nutrient absorption, and overall improved health
- Sense of satisfaction, greater vitality, and a desire to choose better foods and develop better eating habits, permanently

How Does the Body Detoxify Itself?

Keep in mind that detoxification is a continuous process that happens in the body every day all day. We're constantly eliminating toxins through our digestive, urinary, circulatory, respiratory, and lymphatic systems as well as our skin, and they all work well. However, as we get older, they don't function at peak performance due to toxic overload in the body. The body has seven channels of elimination: the blood, the lymphatic system, and five organs—the colon, kidneys, lungs, skin, and liver. All have a unique role to play in getting rid of toxins and wastes, and all must be functioning optimally for effective total-body cleansing. However, the toxic overload in the body means these organs and systems may require assistance to meet the extra demand we put on them.

Let's take a look at the major detoxification organs and systems in the body.

• Colon: The colon is about six feet long and is the part of the body's digestive system that moves waste material from the small intestine to the rectum. The small intestine sucks all the nutrients out of what you eat and then passes the leftover waste to the large intestine. As the colon transports the waste material toward the rectum, it absorbs water from the waste. It may also absorb harmful materials. The longer it takes for waste to pass through the colon, the greater the chance of absorbing such harmful materials back into the body. This is why it is important to have regular, daily bowel movements to keep waste moving out of the body.

• Kidneys: The kidneys, which are located on either side of the lower back, are responsible for filtering the blood in the body and removing materials that the body does not require. These wastes and extra water become urine, which flows to the bladder for release.

• Lungs: Each day, you take about 23,000 breaths, which bring almost 10,000 quarts of air into your lungs. The air that you breathe in contains several gases, including oxygen, which your cells need to function. With each breath, your lungs add fresh oxygen to your blood, which then carries it to your cells.

• Skin: The skin, as the largest organ of the body, is one of our most efficient detoxification organs. Although the liver and kidneys are the primary sources of detoxification, the skin definitely plays an important role as well. When the body is detoxing properly, the skin excretes water and toxins, salt, and other chemicals from our body via sweat. The glands that are connected to millions of tiny hair follicles found in the pores of our skin produce sweat, allowing toxins to be released. We can monitor the state of our overall health by the skin. When our skin has a healthy glow and it's soft to the touch, it indicates that our body is detoxifying properly. In contrast, when our skin has dry patches, acne, hives, and rashes, it indicates that our internal organs are becoming overwhelmed with toxins.

• Liver: The liver, which is the largest of the internal organs, has the most important and comprehensive jobs of all the organs. It has a filtering capacity of one quart of blood every minute, and it has unique metabolic functions. As blood flows through the liver, the detoxification process begins. The liver excretes its toxins in the bile. The bile that is produced by the liver is stored in the gallbladder. It then empties the toxins into the small intestine, and they are eventually eliminated through the colon. However, if you are constipated, these toxins and bile may remain in the intestines too long. This causes toxic poisons that should be eliminated from the body to actually be reabsorbed into the body. These toxins can be stored for months or even years, but they can also be released when you perspire, like with exercise or in a sauna, which are excellent ways to excrete toxins through the skin. There will be much more discussion on the liver later in this section.

• Lymphatic system: The lymphatic system is a secondary circulatory system that supports detoxification and the immune system. The lymphatic system transports toxins and excess fluid, and our sweat glands release toxins through the skin. As tissues become filled with toxins from normal bodily functions, our bodies remove them by carrying them through the bloodstream to be processed by the liver. This occurs through the lymphatic system, which also transports fats and fatty acids as well as immune cells. In a healthy body, the lymphatic system works smoothly and efficiently, but once the body is overloaded with toxins, the lymphatic system can get backed up. Signs that the lymphatic system is working improperly are swelling in the hands, feet, and legs, and cellulite—yes, cellulite, ladies.

The Primary Organ That Makes You Fat or Skinny

The one secret to losing weight and keeping it off is to keep the liver healthy and operating at peak performance. The liver (also known as the fat-burning organ) is the number-one secret weapon to weight loss. The liver is responsible for breaking down, eliminating, and neutralizing toxins in the body and breaking down fats in the body. The liver, which is about the size of a football and weighs in at about three to five pounds, is the largest single organ in the body. Think of the liver as a washing machine for blood. The liver supports the digestive system, controls blood sugar levels, and regulates fat storage. If poisons or excess fats clog your liver, it can't perform its fat-burning function. When your liver cannot metabolize well, you have no energy, you won't absorb nutrients essential for your body to live, and your body can't fight disease.

The liver is responsible for a large variety of health-promoting functions that restore good health and help to maintain weight loss. The liver has all of the following functions:

• It filters your blood to remove toxins such as viruses, bacteria, yeast, and other poisonous foreign substances. When the liver is performing optimally, it can clear 99 percent of toxins from the blood before that blood is distributed to the rest of the body.

• It metabolizes fats by producing bile, a substance that breaks down fats so they can be digested. Daily, your liver produces about a quart of bile, which helps to digest dietary fats by breaking them down so they can be used as fuel.

• It metabolizes carbohydrates and helps the body maintain healthy levels of blood sugar.

• It breaks down proteins into their amino acid parts, creating vital blood proteins.

• It acts as a large storage unit, housing an abundance of substances, including glycogen for stored energy, iron, blood, and vitamins A, D, and B12.

• It keeps your metabolic engines running and your body free of toxins, removing drugs, chemicals, and hormones from the blood—deactivating and eliminating them.

In today's environment, we take in more and more toxins every day: pollutants, birth control pills, prescription medications, household cleaners, food additives, and pesticides. As we age, toxins build up in our system and create a toxic overload in the body. When the liver is overloaded with toxins, it has a difficult time eliminating them, so it begins to store them in fat cells. The more toxins we take in over time, the more fat cells are created in the body. When your liver functions efficiently, it is much easier for you to lose weight. The liver has to perform well enough to eliminate the toxins that are causing fat cells in the body. If you have body fat accumulation, especially around the waist and midsection (i.e., belly fat), it suggests that your liver may not be functioning properly or as efficiently as it could. To lose this excess weight, you have to detoxify and cleanse the liver, which leads to not only a slimmer waistline but also a thinner body.

The most common liver disease in America is a condition known as fatty liver disease, in which the liver stops processing fat and begins storing it right around the waistline. Fatty liver disease affects 20 percent of the population. The major cause of fatty liver disease is overconsumption of sugar, high-fructose corn syrup, and refined carbohydrates (like white flour, white rice, and white sugar). Excess sugar also damages the mitochondria. Mitochondria are the tiny power producers within each cell that convert sugar into energy. As we age, mitochondria become less numerous and less efficient. Each cell has over 1,000 mitochondria when you are young, but less than half that number by the time you are fifty. This means your body produces less energy, resulting in a slower metabolism. One of the principal reasons we gain weight as we age is that our bodies produce less energy, yet we continue to have the same energy intake from food. A fatty liver is also an inflamed liver, producing more inflammatory molecules throughout the body, which leads to more mitochondrial damage. Preventing mitochondrial damage is critical to sustaining weight loss. When the mitochondria are damaged, we can't effectively burn fat or calories, resulting in a slower metabolism and more weight gain.

I know, you might be thinking, I believe my liver is working just fine. But how do you know? Some of the symptoms of toxic overload in the body include bloating, constipation, indigestion, low energy, fatigue, brain fog, depression, weight gain, chronic pain, infections, allergies, and headaches. In the previous section, you can take the "How Toxic Are You?" quiz to assess the toxic overload in your body. If you have concerns about your liver, there are also blood tests that can tell you how well your liver is functioning. However, such tests cannot show the true extent of your liver's functional capacity. In other words, a slight loss in liver function might not show up in traditional blood screening tests. This type of slowdown is often called a "sluggish liver."

- Signs of a sluggish liver are:
- Poor skin tone or flushed facial appearance
- Discoloration of the eyes

- Dark circles
- Yellow-coated tongue
- Acne or breakouts around the nose, cheeks, and chin
- Bitter taste in the mouth
- Headaches
- Moodiness and irritability
- Excessive sweating
- Excessive facial blood vessels
- Red palms and soles, which may also be itchy and inflamed

Although there are several organs of elimination in the body, most health practitioners will agree that the liver is the primary organ of detoxification. It has been said that the length and quality of life depends on proper liver function. Cleansing and detoxification are great for restoring balance in the digestive tract and restoring good liver function. Thus, one of the most important organs to cleanse is the liver. The liver works day and night to cleanse your blood of toxins such as chemicals, poisons, bacteria, and other foreign substances. It is critical to keep it healthy and working at peak performance. There are so many things we do every day that put extra stress on the liver. Things that make it difficult for the liver to eliminate toxins and break down fats are sugar, artificial sweeteners, alcohol, over-the-counter pain relievers, and medications. The liver has to be very healthy to be able to process these substances that are chemical/foreign or unnatural to the body. When the body is overloaded with these toxins, it just stores them in fat cells. In the DHEMM System, we will focus heavily on detoxifying and optimizing liver function.

In summary, the liver breaks down everything that enters your body and distinguishes between the nutrients you need to absorb and the dangerous or unnecessary toxic substances that must be filtered out of your blood. It breaks down foods, beverages, prescription medicines, vitamins, even pesticides from foods. But when the liver is clogged and overwhelmed with toxins, it can't do a very effective job of breaking down foods and processing nutrients and fats. So, if you're concerned with managing your weight, remember this important point: The more toxic your body becomes, the more difficulty you'll have losing weight and keeping it off.

Twelve Ways to Detoxify the Body

Detoxifying the body can be accomplished through various detoxification methods that we'll discuss in detail below. I would encourage you to pick two or three methods to include as a part of your overall health and wellness goals. When you begin detoxifying the body, you may notice a change for the better in your health and energy levels within a few days; however, for others, it may take a few months. Everyone's toxic overload is different, and many factors come into play, such as your health status, weight, metabolism, age, and genetics. So be patient and remain steadfast throughout the detoxification process.

The twelve best ways to effectively detoxify and cleanse the body are listed below.

1. Colon-cleansing herbs/supplements
2. Colonics
3. Liver-cleansing herbs/supplements
4. Foods that detoxify the body
5. Saunas
6. Bikram yoga
7. Detox foot pads/detox foot bath
8. Alkaline water
9. Body brushing
10. Light physical activity
11. Castor oil packs
12. The Master Cleanse

I have used each one of these detox methods on numerous occasions and perform my personal favorites on a weekly basis. You should think of detoxification as a regular, ongoing activity that will help you stay healthy and slim.

- Colon-Cleansing Herbs/Supplements

Colon-cleansing herbs have been used safely for centuries and work a little slower than colonics to detoxify the body but in time achieve good results. They come in the form of powdered or capsule supplements. Their purpose is to force the colon to expel its contents. A benefit of colon cleansing is the reduction of constipation. A poor diet that deprives someone of essential nutrients can cause the intestinal walls to become lined with a plaque-like substance that is not at all good for health.

Colon cleansing not only helps remove the junk from intestinal walls, it also allows waste to pass off more freely. The other noticeable benefit is the elimination of diarrhea. It is a particular condition that is normally caused by toxins, which can cause problems for the whole process of solidifying the waste.

A very powerful and effective colon cleanser that I've used for overnight results is a magnesium-oxygen supplement. It combines magnesium oxide compounds that have been ozonated and stabilized to release oxygen over twelve hours or more throughout the entire digestive system. The magnesium acts as a vehicle to transport the oxygen throughout the body and has the gentle effect of loosening toxins and acidic waste and transporting them out of the body. Oxygen also supports the growth of friendly bacteria, which is essential for proper digestive and intestinal health. For intensive colon cleansing, magnesium-oxygen supplements taken for seven to ten days are an effective way to jump-start a detoxification program.

They are safe for regular use and can also be used on a longer-term basis for daily, ongoing detoxification. In contrast to synthetic laxatives, a quality magnesium-oxygen supplement is non-habit-forming and actually strengthens all the organs' functions, making it a safe, long-term option. As always, check with your doctor and be sure to follow the directions on the label. For most people, anywhere from three to five supplements taken at bedtime for seven to ten days will provide an effective colon cleansing. If you experience loose stools or other side effects, simply reduce the dosage and be sure to take just once a day.

Magnesium-oxygen supplements are safe for regular use, but I would recommend they be used only periodically during heavy detoxification and cleansing to help keep the colon clean and increase bowel activity.

Different herbs perform different actions and therefore produce different results, so it's important to know what goal you would like to achieve when choosing your herbal colon-cleansing product. Some work like a laxative to help you eliminate fecal matter and prevent toxic buildup; others kill harmful bacteria and parasites; others soften the stool, add bulk, and improve the function of colon muscles to promote healthy and regular bowel movements. So if you want a product that works strictly as a laxative, you will make a different choice than someone who wants to add bulk and clean out the colon or kill parasites. Please watch the stool to see what comes out. You will be amazed, and possibly disgusted.

- Colonics

A colonic, also known as colon hydrotherapy, is a method used to remove waste and impacted fecal matter from the colon. The first modern colonic machine was invented about a hundred years ago. Today, colonic hygienists or colon therapists perform colonics. Colonics work somewhat like an enema but involve much more water and none of the odors or discomfort. While you lie on a table, a machine or gravity-driven pump slowly flushes up to 20 gallons of water through a tube inserted into the rectum. After the water is in the colon, the therapist may massage your abdomen. Then the therapist flushes out the fluids and waste through another tube. The therapist may repeat the process. A session may last up to an hour. The therapist may use a variety of water pressures and temperatures.

The average colon weighs up to four pounds, but it is not unusual at all for colon cleansing to flush away as much as ten to twenty pounds of stagnant fecal matter. Your colon can hold a great deal of waste material that, when not eliminated, putrefies, adding to the toxic load of your body.

Many people with "potbellies" may actually have several pounds of old, hardened fecal matter lodged within their colons. As a result, the process will actually cause you to experience some immediate weight loss. It is a common misconception that doing a colonic will cause your body to get rid of all the good and bad bacteria. If you decide to do a colonic, it will rinse out good bacteria in your colon—but just temporarily. After you flush out everything, the good bacteria with the bad, you want to replace the good bacteria, the probiotics. Your body will replenish the good bacteria within twenty-four hours, unless you are extremely unhealthy or weak. However, you should always take a probiotic supplement after a colonic to replenish the good bacteria right away. A good colon therapist will always provide you with probiotics (good bacteria) at the end of your colonics session.

If you choose to research colonics and decide to include them as part of your detoxification process, you probably want to go at least once a week for up to six weeks, particularly when you first begin aggressively detoxifying the body. That is because you are drawing out toxins in the body, and if they are not eliminated quickly, they can cause detox symptoms that become uncomfortable. One rule of thumb as to whether to do a colonic is determined by how frequent your bowel movements are. If your body is managing the toxins and waste well through normal daily bowel movements (one to two per day), then you probably don't need to have a colonic. If your bowel movements are less frequent than once a day, it may be a good idea to do a colonic to get your bowels moving more frequently. There are no major drawbacks to a properly administered colonic by a trained colon hydrotherapist. You don't need to be concerned about the safety of colonics as long as they're done with a certified colon therapist on a good-quality machine.

Here is another simple way to evaluate your health. As an example, bowel movements (BMs) that are black or reddish indicate potential health problems. Thin BMs suggest that more fiber is needed in the diet or there is some type of imbalance in the digestive tract. If you have chronic constipation and your BMs are rock solid, this may be an indication that your liver is overworked. If you experience chronic constipation or difficult bowel movements for an extended period of time, you should seek medical advice.

Your bowel movements will help you understand what's going on with your body. Healthy bowel movements should:

- Occur two to three times a day and definitely no less than once per day
- Not have a strong, foul odor
- Be medium brown in color, shaped like a banana, about the width of a sausage
- Be 4 to 8 inches long and should enter the water smoothly and slowly fall once it reaches the water

These guidelines should help you check your poop to constantly evaluate the overall health of your digestive system and toxic overload in your body.

- Liver Cleansing Herbs/Supplements

Earlier in this section, we discussed how important the liver was to losing weight and staying healthy. The liver is responsible for breaking down and eliminating toxins in the body, as well as breaking down fats in the body. Therefore, it is essential that we cleanse the liver to improve the body's detoxification capabilities and to help the body metabolize and burn fats. One easy way to cleanse the liver is to take herbs/supplements, such as milk thistle, dandelion root, and burdock. These herbs are all-natural and very effective at liver detoxification. You'll find that many products on the market combine these herbs into one supplement so that you can achieve the best results. As you look for products to help you cleanse your liver, be sure to only use those that are all-natural and gentle on the body. Completing a liver cleanse can be a positive and rejuvenating experience and yield numerous health benefits. As you improve liver health, you increase your body's ability to detoxify itself, improve its fat-burning capabilities, and achieve optimum health.

Foods That Detoxify the Body

When you eat natural, organic healthy foods, you keep your insides clean and begin to look radiant despite your age. When you eat more natural, raw foods, you simply look and feel better. Foods and herbs that detoxify and cleanse the body are:

• Green leafy veggies: When you are ready to detox your body, fill your refrigerator with kale, wheatgrass, spinach, spirulina, alfalfa, chard, arugula, and other organic leafy greens. These veggies are even better for cleansing the body when they are eaten raw or juiced raw in a juicer. These plants will help give a chlorophyll boost to your digestive tract. Chlorophyll rids the body of harmful environmental toxins from smog, heavy metals, herbicides, cleaning products, and pesticides. Green leafy veggies are also high in naturally occurring sulfur and glutathione, which help the liver detoxify harmful chemicals.

• Onions: Onions, scallions (green onions), and shallots are sources of sulfur-containing amino acids. According to Patrick Holford and Fiona McDonald Joyce, authors of the book The 9-Day Liver Detox Diet, sulfur drives a critical liver-detox pathway known as sulfation. The amino acids present in onions provide the raw materials to make glutathione, a detoxifying compound in the liver. Glutathione detoxifies acetaminophen and caffeine that pass through the organ. These authors recommend eating a small onion, a shallot, or four green onions raw every day to garner the full detoxifying effect. Raw red onions are particularly beneficial as they contain quercetin, a natural antiinflammatory that enhances liver function.

• Citrus fruits (grapefruits, lemons, limes, and oranges): These citrus wonders aid the body in flushing out toxins as well as jump-starting the digestive tract with enzymatic processes. They also aid the liver in its cleansing processes. To increase detoxification, start each morning with a warm glass of lemon water. Remember, vitamin C is a great detoxification vitamin, as it transforms toxins into digestible material.

• Broccoli sprouts: Broccoli sprouts are extremely high in antioxidants and can help stimulate the detoxification enzymes in the digestive tract like no other vegetable. The sprouts are actually more effective than the fully grown vegetable.

• Garlic: This pungent bulb stimulates the liver to produce detoxification enzymes that help filter out toxic residues in the digestive system. Adding sliced or cooked garlic to any dish will help aid any detox diet.

• Seeds and nuts: Incorporate more of the easily digestible seeds and nuts into your diet. These include flaxseed, pumpkin seeds, almonds, walnuts, hemp seeds, sesame seeds, chia seeds, Siberian cedar nuts, and sunflower seeds.

• Omega-3 oils: Use hemp oil, avocado oil, olive oil, fish oil, or flaxseed oil while detoxing. These will help lubricate the intestinal walls, allowing the toxins to be absorbed by the oil and eliminated by the body.

• Beans: Eat plenty of beans. Beans contain the potent enzyme cholecystokinin, which naturally suppresses your appetite while providing protein to your liver to help detox your body. Add beans to your meals easily by adding them to your salad or just eating them as a side dish.

• Green tea: Packed full of antioxidants, green tea not only washes toxins out of the system through its liquid content, it also contains a special type of antioxidant, called catechins, known to increase liver function.

• Green smoothies.

• Saunas

The skin is the largest organ of elimination for the body, and a sauna helps you sweat out toxins from the body. I love the sauna because I'm all about things that have a health benefit while providing a beauty benefit. You can kill two birds with one stone. You release toxins, burn calories, and come out with glowing skin. I personally love getting in the sauna. I had a client who learned about saunas from my teleseminars and found that after using the sauna, her acne cleared up; she was sweating out the toxins instead of letting them clog up her pores. If you want to know how healthy someone is, sometimes you can just look at his or her skin and tell. If someone has clear, radiant skin, there's a good chance he or she is very healthy; breakouts, puffiness, or dry skin indicate that the body is having some health problems. Experts say that a sauna session can do more to clean, detoxify, and simply "freshen" your skin than anything else.

Benefits of the Sauna:

• Weight loss: Burn 300 to 500 calories in fifteen to twenty minutes, almost equivalent to one to two hours of brisk walking or one hour of exercise. Saunas works positively on metabolism, increasing its speed and intensity, which in turn results in weight loss.

• Elimination of toxins: Steam saunas induce perspiration, which is how the body purges itself of toxins and impurities. The heat of the steam causes the body's temperature to rise, which can help kill any virus, bacteria, fungus, or parasite in the body.

• Improved skin: Steam opens up the pores of the skin, allowing impurities and toxins to flush themselves out of the body. The steam also hydrates and moisturizes the skin, making steam saunas particularly beneficial to people with dry skin.

• Strengthened immune system: The steam in a steam sauna opens up the pores, allowing the skin to sweat out toxins that can cause illness. The high temperature of a steam sauna causes an artificial fever, which sends a "wake-up call" to the immune system and increases an individual's white blood cell count.

• Relaxed muscles: The heat from the steam warms and relaxes tense muscles. This relaxation helps to reduce stress levels, revive mental clarity, and improve overall physical and emotional health.

For a steam sauna, you sit in moist heat for fifteen to twenty minutes. Follow that with a quick shower to wash off all of the toxins that have been flushed from your skin and to feel truly refreshed. Another type of sauna is an infrared sauna, which produces what is known as radiant heat. The heat of an infrared sauna also penetrates more deeply without the discomfort and draining effect often experienced in a conventional steam sauna. An infrared sauna produces two to three times more sweat volume, and due to the lower temperatures used (110° to 130°F), it is considered a safer alternative for those at cardiovascular risk. It accelerates the removal of toxic wastes and chemicals that are stored and lodged in the fatty tissues of the body. The sweating caused by deep heat helps eliminate dead skin cells and improve skin tone and elasticity. The heat produced in infrared saunas is extremely helpful for various skin conditions, including acne, eczema, and cellulite. Another benefit of the sauna is that you burn calories. Studies have shown that you can burn 600 calories in thirty minutes in an infrared sauna. Whichever you prefer, steam or infrared sauna, both can be dehydrating, so it is important to hydrate properly before and after a sauna.

- Bikram Yoga

I once heard that doing Bikram yoga for detoxification is one of the best ways to rid your body of unwanted wastes and toxins. Now that I have done Bikram yoga, I would definitely agree! During a Bikram yoga class, the body removes toxic waste through the skin via sweat, as your skin is one of the largest waste-disposal systems in the body. On its own, yoga is already a powerful fitness regimen because you work out every muscle in the body, making them all strong and flexible. In the ninety-minute Bikram yoga class, there are twenty-six poses performed, along with two breathing exercises. The poses are performed in a room with temperatures reaching between 95° and 100°F. At high temperatures, you will begin to sweat profusely, allowing the toxic waste to be removed from the body. This allows your skin to convert toxins that come from various fats into simpler, more water-soluble compounds that can be easily removed. It has been reported that you actually burn 750 to 900 calories in a ninety minute Bikram yoga session. As an added benefit, you get to learn the techniques of meditation, which can help you relax your mind and alleviate stress. Bikram yoga is an effective means to achieving balance among mind, body, and spirit.

- Detox Foot Pads/Detox Foot Bath

Detox foot pads are a quick and easy way to rid the body of toxins. You put the pads on the bottoms of your feet overnight as you sleep. The ingredients in the detox foot pads are said to pull impurities and toxins out of your system during the night while you sleep. In the morning, you remove the pads from your feet and discard them. They are helpful with aches, pains, sore muscles, joint pains, swelling, and bloating. The detox foot bath (ionic foot bath) works by soaking your feet in a warm saltwater solution made up of many different toxin-drawing ingredients. The ionic activity in the water shoots through your body fat and is supposed to draw the toxins out through the hundreds of pores in your feet.

- Alkaline Water

Drinking alkaline water (ion water or hydrogen-rich water) detoxifies the body and leaves the skin looking smoother, more elastic, and more youthful. The benefits of drinking alkaline water are detoxification, better hydration, and increased energy. Some brands of alkaline bottled water include Blue Delta and Essential Water. You can buy a portable alkaline water bottle (e.g., IonPod) that converts regular water to alkaline water or buy an expensive machine that converts the water from your faucet to alkaline water (such as Kangen Water). It is recommended that you don't drink alkaline water with food or within thirty minutes before or after meals. You also want to build up how much alkaline water your body can handle, beginning with about eight ounces a day. If you drink too much alkaline water too quickly, you will get strong detox symptoms, such as headaches or rashes.

- Body Brushing

Body brushing (also known as dry brushing) is done with a natural boarbristle brush, which can be found in health food stores, Whole Foods, or Trader Joe's. Dry brushing on a regular basis lightens the burden on the liver by helping to remove excess waste from the body. Dry brushing stimulates the lymphatic system, which is a secondary circulatory system underneath the skin that rids the body of toxic wastes, bacteria, and dead cells. By body brushing, you move the toxins along and out of the body for elimination. By brushing the body from head to toe with the dry brush, focusing on the lymphatic drainage regions, like behind the knee, you'll improve the efficiency of the whole lymphatic system. Firm, gentle brushstrokes across the skin will improve your blood circulation, clean out clogged pores, and enable your body to remove toxins faster. Body brushing removes dead skin layers and encourages cell renewal for smoother skin. If the liver is the fat-burning organ, then the lymph system can be called a fat-processing system. So cleansing the liver and lymphatic system are key to weight loss and diminishing cellulite.

To effectively use the body brush, first remove your clothes. Begin brushing the soles of the feet. Next, brush from the ankles to the calves, concentrating on the area behind the knees, using long upward, firm strokes toward the heart. Then brush from the knees to the groin, the thighs, and the buttocks. If you're a woman, make circular strokes around your thighs and buttocks to help mobilize fat stores, such as cellulite. (Dry brushing actually helps to diminish cellulite.) Then brush the torso, avoiding the breasts. Finally, make long strokes from the wrists to the shoulders and underarms. The entire process should take no more than three to five minutes and will leave your skin feeling totally invigorated. The best times to brush are in the morning before showering or at night before you go to bed.

- Light Physical Activity

Just by doing mild or light physical activity, you oxygenate your body to protect it against toxic overload. Simple movements increase the oxygen content of your blood and dissolve and help to wash out sludge that accumulates in and on your arteries; in other words, it cleanses waste from your bloodstream. For example, as little as thirty minutes of brisk walking can prompt this type of cleansing.

- Castor Oil Packs

Castor oil packs are typically used by naturopaths to help stimulate and detoxify the liver. A castor oil pack is placed directly on the skin to increase circulation and to promote elimination of toxins and healing of the tissues and organs underneath the skin. It is used to stimulate the liver, relieve pain, increase lymphatic circulation, reduce inflammation, and improve digestion. Castor oil packs are made by soaking a piece of cotton or wool flannel in castor oil and placing it on the abdomen and especially over the liver. The flannel is covered with a sheet of plastic wrap, and a hot water bottle or heating pad is placed over the plastic to heat the pack. You keep the pack on for thirty to forty-five minutes while in a relaxed position. Rest while the pack is in place but do not fall asleep and leave the heating pad on all night.

After removing the pack, cleanse the area with a solution of water and baking soda. Store the pack in a covered container in the refrigerator. Each pack may be reused up to thirty times. It is generally recommended that a castor oil pack be used for three to seven days in one week as a detoxification treatment. You can place the cloth on the right side of the abdomen to stimulate the liver or directly on inflamed and swollen joints and muscle strains. It can be used on the abdomen to relieve constipation and other digestive disorders and on the lower abdomen in cases of menstrual irregularities and uterine and ovarian cysts. Castor oil should not be taken internally. It should not be applied to broken skin or used during pregnancy, breastfeeding, or during menstrual flow.

- The Master Cleanse

The Master Cleanse is an advanced detoxification method, and it's a great way to jump-start weight loss. It cleans out the accumulated fats in your tissues and liver while purging excess fluid buildup from your system. The Master Cleanse is designed to support all the organs involved in detoxification—the liver, kidney, lungs, lymphatic system, colon, and skin. Detoxification diets like the Master Cleanse have crossed into the mainstream and are often marketed as a quick and easy way to lose weight. However, the Master Cleanse is not a weight-loss system; rather, it's a way to detoxify and cleanse the body, restoring it to great health. View the Master Cleanse as a stepping-stone to a healthier lifestyle. In fact, if you decide to do the Master Cleanse, once you complete the ten days, you should transition to eating healthier, natural foods so that you do not gain all the weight back. The Master Cleanse accelerates fat loss from fat-storage areas like the hips, thighs, belly, and buttocks. It will transform your body, with the focus on losing inches as opposed to pounds. However, many people do report losing up to fifteen pounds in ten days. Fat cells shrink as excess toxins stored in them are purged from your body, ensuring that you are losing fat, bloat, and water weight but not muscle.

The first phase requires that you eat no solid foods for ten days. Instead, you ingest a "lemonade" drink that cleanses the body, provides fuel, and prevents hunger. You will take in about 1,000 to 1,200 calories a day. This lighter caloric load allows the body to better metabolize and process toxins and remove them from the body. The Master Cleanse is not actually a complete fast, as you consume up to 1,200 calories each day, depending upon how much of the lemonade drink you have throughout the day. The detox fast is designed to keep you energized enough to work and enjoy your daily activities. As a matter of fact, since detox fasting increases the body's detoxification capabilities, you may end up experiencing more energy after several days on it.

There are many benefits to the Master Cleanse, such as providing a rest to the digestive system. Your body uses a significant amount of your energy every day in digesting, absorbing, and assimilating your food, so the Master Cleanse gives your digestive tract a chance to rest and repair. This, in turn, gives your overworked liver a chance to catch up on its function of detoxification. During fasting, the cells, tissues, and organs expel accumulated wastes, helping cells heal, repair, and strengthen. The Master Cleanse is helpful because it cleanses the liver, the body's key fat-burning organ, and allows it to rest, improving its ability to break down fats more efficiently and operate at peak performance. The Master Cleanse provides the added benefit of improving your appearance by deep cleansing every cell in your body; your skin will glow with radiance, and the whites of your eyes will become clearer and whiter and may even sparkle. You will feel and look better than you have in years. Your energy will be supercharged. The Master Cleanse rejuvenates the body physically, mentally, and spiritually.

Some people should not do the Master Cleanse. They are:

• People who are undergoing chemotherapy or who have completed chemotherapy within the last six months.

• People who are recovering from major surgery or a severe wound or injury.

• Children in their growing years (under the age of eighteen).

• Pregnant or nursing women. Pregnancy is not a time to detoxify the body but to provide nourishment for the body.

• People allergic to "everything" or who have frequent allergy symptoms.

• The obese (more than seventy pounds overweight).

• People in poor general health.

• People with a multi-year history of taking strong medical or psychiatric drugs.

• Those who use medication for chronic health conditions, such as diabetes, heart disease, high blood pressure, or high cholesterol.

• Anyone with cancer or a terminal illness.

• Anyone with kidney failure or borderline kidney function (best identified by your doctor through blood tests).

• Ten Ways to Detoxify Your Home

To help minimize toxins in your home and environment, follow these tips:

1. Don't smoke or allow smoking inside your home or car.

2. Leave all shoes at the door as opposed to bringing them into your living quarters.

3. Avoid or air out dry cleaning. Use an organic dry cleaner. If you don't have one near you and feel you must use your local dry cleaner, let your newly dry-cleaned clothes air out in the garage or on the porch for a few days before bringing them into the house.

4. Use unscented laundry detergent and fabric softener.

5. Don't use air fresheners that contain solvents.

6. Replace your furnace filters every six weeks with high-quality pleated filters rated a minimum efficiency reporting value (MERV) of 7 to 9.

7. Buy an air purifier that has both charcoal and high-efficiency particulate air filters for your bedroom.

8. Use tile flooring or real wood flooring instead of carpeting.

9. Ensure that there is no mold overgrowth anywhere in your home.

10. Install a chlorine filter on your showerhead; this will also help you have softer hair and skin as well.

If, despite your best efforts, you have still failed when it comes to losing weight and keeping it off, it's most likely because you've missed an important key to losing weight permanently: getting the toxins out of the body. One of my clients sent me a note saying, "Thanks for the great detoxification tips, they are working; I haven't even changed the way I eat, and already I've lost thirteen pounds by your cleansing and detoxification tips." I get this quite often. Once you start cleansing, you become more aware of how your body feels after eating certain foods and drinks. You start paying closer attention to what you eat. You start to recognize what nurtures and nourishes the body and what does not. You begin to let go of emotional toxins along with the physical toxins. You begin to let go of people, places, things, and emotions that are harmful and do not nourish the mind and body.

You've often heard people say, "Calories in, calories out." But from now on, the phrase in your mind should be, "Clean the gut, lose the gut" or "Toxins out, weight off." It is possible to overcome genetics and win the battle of the bulge. It is possible to help your body eliminate toxic wastes that slow down your metabolism, throw off your hormonal balance, and cause you to gain weight.

Correct Hormonal Imbalances

We all know that fad diets are a thing of the past. The mantra "eat less and exercise more" is ineffective for many people who want to lose weight. We know that the no-carb, low-carb, no-fat, low-fat crazes of the eighties and nineties were hit-or-miss in terms of results. But now, we have better scientific information on one of the more important factors that helps us lose weight: hormonal balance. Welcome to the world of understanding your hormones, the little messengers that control your appetite, metabolism, and how much weight you gain or lose. Please note that if you are a woman over the age of thirty-five, there are three key sex hormones (estrogen, progesterone, and testosterone) that play a role in weight gain.

It is essential to understand how hormones play a role in maintaining our weight. Hormones control almost every aspect of how we gain and lose weight. Some hormones tell you you're hungry, some tell you you're full; some tell your body what to do with the food that is eaten, whether to use it as fuel for energy or store it as fat, which causes us to gain weight. Hormones are responsible for metabolizing fat. By controlling your hormones, you can control your weight.

Hormones affect how you feel, how you look, and, most important, how you maintain your weight and health. When your hormones are balanced properly, you will have great health, beauty, and vibrancy. When your hormones are imbalanced, you have mood swings, you crave unhealthy foods, and you feel sluggish and lethargic. In this section, I will explain which hormones are critical to weight loss, how they work, and how they help you stay slim and healthy. I once had an unexplained weight gain of thirty pounds, practically overnight, in just a few months. If I ate a Big Mac, I gained a pound by the next day. But today I can easily eat 2,000 calories of nutrient-rich foods a day, without exercising, and still maintain my current weight. None of this would be possible without finely tuned hormones that accelerate my metabolism and cause me to burn fat as opposed to storing fat.

When I was in my late thirties, my hormones began to have a mind of their own and made me feel out of control. If you're like me, you've experienced some of the following:

- Adult acne (skin that breaks out more than when you were a teenager)

- Fatigue and low energy, even when you get a good night's sleep
- Eating less and not losing a single pound
- Skin that's sagging and showing fine lines and wrinkles
- Severe mood swings, even when you're not on your cycle
- Unexplained weight gain of ten, twenty, or thirty pounds for no apparent reason—you haven't changed anything in your diet or lifestyle

I knew that something had changed in my body, but initially I didn't understand the effect my hormones had on my metabolism, weight, moods, health, and well-being. Since then, I've studied cutting-edge research about natural ways to balance my hormones and blood sugar levels to support weight loss. Through reading and research, and my studies as a certified nutritionist and weight-management expert, I learned a great deal about endocrinology, the field of medicine that deals with hormones and glands. I was happy to learn that I was not going crazy and that it was hormonal imbalances that were changing the way I felt and how much weight I gained. It was as if a light was turned on and I could finally see a critical aspect of controlling my weight. The more I talked to others, especially women, the more I realized I was not alone. I'm happy to reap the benefits of a stronger metabolism now, but for years my hormones were working against me. I didn't understand much about them years ago, but now I know how to ensure they work in my favor.

Hormones Control Your Appetite

Have you ever thought about what tells your brain when you're hungry or when you're full? One of the major reasons many Americans gain extra weight is that their appetite-control system is out of balance. The various chemical systems and messengers in the body that tell them when they are hungry and when they are full have been disrupted. Rebalancing the chemical hormonal imbalances will get your appetite-control system functioning properly again. There are certain hormones that balance hunger and fullness in the brain that are key to permanent weight control. If you were never hungry, losing weight would be very easy. If you properly control the hormones that are directly affected by what you eat, you will not be hungry between meals and will have sufficient fuel and energy for the day. This will expedite fat loss.

Feeling hungry is one of the most powerful urges we have. When you feel hungry, everything else is secondary to getting food into your system. This is because the brain becomes desperate to get the energy it needs to function. There are hormones that control your weight, often called metabolic hormones, brain messenger chemicals called neuropeptides, and messenger molecules of the immune system called cytokines, produced in the fat cells, white blood cells, and liver cells. All of these components work together to communicate to the organs and tissues responsible for managing your weight and keeping you alive. Good communication results in a healthy metabolism. These finely tuned systems determine your health and metabolism. They are what tell you that you are full and to stop eating, making the difference between whether you gain or lose weight.

Let's see how these complex messenger signals work. When your stomach is empty, one of the chemical messengers secretes hormones that tell your body and brain you are hungry. Your brain then prepares the stomach to receive some food. When you eat, the food enters the gut and your body releases yet more hormones, preparing the food for digestion. As the food makes its way into your bloodstream, more messages coordinate your metabolism, telling your pancreas to produce insulin. Your fat cells then send hormonal messages back to your brain to stop eating, along with signals from your stomach that you are full. Your liver then metabolizes or processes fat and sugar and helps use it for energy or stores the excess as fat.

Your body can't work the way it's supposed to if any one of the hormones is out of sync. You have to be able to naturally optimize how all of your hormones work as opposed to trying to address just one at a time. They are too closely integrated to address one; if one is out of sync, then there are already other chemical imbalances in the body. The reason I say "naturally" is because this book doesn't focus on expensive drugs or other dangerous methods but rather addresses the underlying causes of hormonal imbalances, which are our diet (foods we eat), lifestyle (sleep and stress), and environmental factors (toxins and pollutants).

Six Hormones That Affect Weight Gain

There are six hormones that affect weight, and when they are unbalanced, it will be difficult for you to lose weight. Here is a brief overview of how these six hormones affect weight gain.

- Glucagon

Glucagon is a hormone secreted by the pancreas that raises blood glucose levels. It has the opposite effect of insulin, which lowers blood glucose levels. Without adequate levels of glucagon, you will feel hungry and tired because the brain is not getting enough fuel (blood sugar). It is important to balance insulin and glucagon in the body to maintain blood sugar levels. If insulin makes you store fat, then glucagon helps you burn it. It works in the liver to help regulate both blood sugar and fat usage. Eating protein affects the hormone glucagon, which is why eating protein and carbohydrates together is crucial for maintaining stable blood sugar levels.

- Cortisol

Cortisol is secreted by the adrenal glands and its primary functions are to increase blood sugar and aid in fat, protein, and carbohydrate metabolism. When you are stressed, your body releases cortisol (also known as the stress hormone). Fat caused by stress (i.e., stress fat) stores in the belly. Studies have shown that when cortisol is released into the bloodstream, you become less sensitive to leptin, the hormone that tells your brain you are full. When this happens, you tend to eat more and begin to crave sugar. That means that your body not only slows down your metabolism when you are stressed out, it actually tells you to consume more food. Cortisol can be very good or very bad. If cortisol is released with high insulin levels and low testosterone, it can store fat; and if it is released with large amounts of testosterone, it enhances fat burning.

- Leptin

Leptin is a protein hormone that has a central role in fat metabolism. Leptin is nicknamed the natural appetite suppressant. Leptin controls how hungry you are on a daily basis. When leptin doesn't function properly, it creates an imbalance that results in a slow metabolism, premature aging, and disease. Leptin resistance is a hormonal imbalance that disrupts the body's natural ability to regulate appetite and metabolism. If you become leptin-resistant, you will eat and eat like you're starving. Some people get extremely obese because their bodies never receive the message to stop eating and start burning. Leptin tells your brain when you are full. But when levels are too low, leptin signals your body to store fat. Obviously, you want to keep levels of leptin high in your body, and there are ways to do that naturally. Seafood and fish are known to raise leptin levels because of the omega-3 fatty acids. Omega-3s/fish oil are also available as supplements.

- Thyroid

The thyroid gland is a butterfly-shaped gland located in your neck just below your Adam's apple. Thyroid hormones perform many functions: they help control the amount of oxygen each cell uses, the rate at which the body burns calories, heart rate, body temperature, fertility, digestion, mood, and memory. Thyroid hormones have a profound impact on weight because they regulate how the body burns carbohydrates and fats. Thyroid problems are very common in this country; over 25 million people have some sort of thyroid imbalance. Statistics also show that less than half of them know they have it. When the thyroid is not functioning properly, especially if it becomes underactive, every part of the body is adversely affected. Reduced thyroid activity, or hypothyroidism, causes the metabolic rate to decrease, which greatly affects weight.

- Human Growth Hormone (HGH)

HGH is considered to be a "building" hormone because it sends signals to the body to be lean and muscular and work to ensure fat is burned and not stored. HGH is one of the most talked-about hormones of modern times. By now, you've probably seen infomercials and products praising the benefits of human growth hormone as the fountain of youth. Our HGH naturally starts to decline in our thirties and forties, and lack of HGH activity promotes weight gain, particularly around the waist and midsection. Typically, your body will use blood sugar (glucose) for energy before it taps into fat for energy. What HGH does is force your body to draw energy from your fat reserves first, turning your body into a fat-burning machine, even when you're inactive, resting, or even sleeping. HGH is also known to help your body grow new muscle cells, which is particularly good because your body normally stops making muscle cells after your late teens. So if you do weight or resistance training, HGH will help you get toned muscles. You can naturally boost your HGH levels with certain foods, exercise, and a proper night's rest. Sleep deprivation almost completely destroys HGH production; it is during deep sleep that the body produces HGH.

- Insulin

Insulin is a hormone secreted by the pancreas in response to eating food; its job is to send glucose out of the blood into the tissue cells for use as energy. When excess glucose remains in the blood, insulin levels stay high. Chronically elevated insulin can cause both fat storage and more inflammation in the body. When insulin levels are high, this is a signal to the body to store extra calories as fat and to refrain from burning fat. Because insulin is the hormone most responsible for the obesity epidemic in our country, we will focus on it for the remainder of this section.

Insulin Makes You Fat Even If You're Not Diabetic

One of the primary causes of obesity is the excess production of the hormone insulin. Many specialists have stated that it is excess insulin that makes you fat and keeps you fat. Insulin creates fat in the body by taking sugar and placing it into fat cells. In order to control your weight, you must control your insulin levels.

Many researchers have found that the majority of people with weight problems produce too much insulin. For most overweight people, insulin is the enemy. The bottom line for most people is that to get rid of fat they have to reduce their insulin levels. If they want to reduce insulin, they have to take away sugar. Sugar (i.e., refined, starchy carbohydrates) stimulates insulin production. And as we've learned from many diet books, reducing carbohydrates is a must. Low-carb diets are initially effective for overweight people because carbohydrates cause the overproduction of insulin, and by cutting out carbs, this overproduction of insulin stops.

However, the key thing to understand is why the body produces too much insulin in the first place. It is due to a hormonal imbalance, which once corrected, will stop the overproduction of insulin in the body. The problem with the low-carb diets is that once you go off those diets, you just gain the weight right back. However, my approach goes further in that it addresses the underlying reason as to why the body is producing too much insulin. Eating fewer carbohydrates helps reduce insulin spikes, but correcting the reason why you produce too much insulin will allow you to address your weight issues once and for all.

Carbohydrates, a key element of the human diet, are abundant in fruits, grains, breads, pastas, cereals, rice, and potatoes. Carbohydrates are the body's primary source of energy. Carbohydrates are broken down during digestion into a sugar known as glucose. Glucose, the simplest sugar, is the only one that the body can use for energy; every one of the body's cells needs glucose in order to function. The amount of glucose in your blood is also called your blood glucose level. A normal glucose level in the blood is 80 to 100 mg/dl.

Now, here's where insulin comes into play. Insulin is a powerful hormone that regulates the glucose levels in the blood. When you have more glucose in your body than your cells need, insulin takes the extra and stores it as fat in the body, allowing your blood glucose levels to return to normal. Thus, insulin regulates blood glucose levels. But when those insulin levels are too high, it begins storing fat in the body. High insulin levels mean you'll have more body fat, while low insulin levels mean you'll have less body fat. Carbohydrates are the foods that cause these insulin spikes that result in excess fat in the body. When you always have unusually high levels of blood glucose in the body, you have a condition known as diabetes, which is potentially very damaging to the body. Insulin not only regulates blood sugar levels, it also triggers a biological switch that turns off the production of muscle and turns on the production of fat, particularly around the waist and belly area. That's why you'll often hear insulin called the fat-storage hormone. Insulin also interferes with the breakdown of fat cells, making it even more difficult for your body to lose weight.

What Is Insulin Resistance?

If you have tried different popular diets, counted calories, eaten smaller portions, and exercised but still have been struggling to lose weight no matter what you tried, you may be one of the growing number of people who suffer from a hormone condition known as "insulin resistance." It is believed that 75 percent of Americans have this condition. It is also not uncommon for those who suffer from it to have other health issues, including high blood pressure, high cholesterol, and sometimes diabetes. If you have insulin resistance, you can correct both your weight gain and your health issues through the DHEMM System. Insulin resistance is extremely common: three out of four people have it. But the majority of them don't even know it. I will help you discover if you have insulin resistance and if it's the problem behind your inability to lose weight. You'll be pleased to learn how eating clean and balanced foods help you lose weight if you are insulin resistant. You'll also learn how to combine certain foods to help you lose weight and avoid foods that will cause you to gain weight. You'll see improvements in other health-related issues, including the lowering of high blood pressure and high cholesterol as well.

Insulin resistance, also known as metabolic syndrome, prediabetes, or syndrome X, is a genetic condition that makes it difficult for you to lose weight because your body overreacts to foods that are high in carbohydrates. As a certified nutritionist, I have a great understanding of the science of foods and how foods affect our ability to lose or gain weight. Since I also suffer from insulin resistance, I am personally knowledgeable as to which foods aggravate my condition and cause me to gain weight and feel sluggish and tired. How you eat and what foods you combine are essential to managing insulin resistance and maintaining permanent weight loss. Each time you eat a high-carbohydrate food or sugar, your blood sugar levels rise, and in response, your body releases insulin to get rid of the excess blood sugar. However, the more your pancreas secretes insulin to control blood sugar, the less sensitive or responsive your body becomes to insulin. In other words, your body becomes resistant to insulin. So then, your body has to secrete even more insulin to lower your blood sugar levels. This creates insulin resistance.

Pure sugars, such as sucrose and high-fructose corn syrups, are digested very quickly, which leads to a rapid increase in blood sugar levels. Additionally, certain carbohydrates, such as breads, bagels, muffins, pizza, pasta, and potatoes, are also digested quickly. When blood sugar levels rise very quickly, the body responds with a surge of insulin. This surge leads to excess fat storage in the body while also making you hungrier due to the extreme ups and downs in glucose and insulin levels. If you are insulin-resistant and eat high-carbohydrate foods, you will produce up to four times more insulin than normal just to be able to bring your blood glucose levels back to normal, healthy levels. I was not surprised to learn that the body can begin storing fat in as little as two hours after eating a high-carbohydrate meal or food, as I had often felt that after a large pasta dinner, I had gained one or two pounds by morning. The good news about the DHEMM System is that I teach you how to eat clean and balanced foods to keep your insulin levels from spiking so that you can lose weight and stay slim.

What Causes Insulin Resistance?

Some people have higher-than-normal insulin levels and others do not. People who have higher-than-normal insulin levels are considered insulin resistant. This condition causes their body to overreact to carbohydrates by causing higher-than-normal insulin spikes, causing them to get fat faster than people who don't have insulin resistance. The difficult part is that as your body begins to store fat, you become even more insulin resistant, resulting in even more weight gain. People who consume a great deal of refined, starchy carbohydrates, such as breads, muffins, pasta, potatoes, noodles, and bagels, and sweets, such as cakes, pies, pastries, sodas, sweetened juice, and sugary cereals, have an increased risk of developing insulin resistance. All of these foods cause blood sugar levels to rise and fall rapidly, causing the body to secrete more and more insulin to lower blood sugar levels.

Certain other substances also increase insulin levels, such as caffeine, artificial sweeteners, and nicotine. You may think that your diet soda with an artificial sweetener is relatively harmless because it has no calories and will not raise blood glucose levels, but it will cause insulin levels to rise, contributing to your insulin resistance symptoms. Our goal is to avoid spikes in blood sugar, which trigger insulin release and lead to the storing of fat! To determine if you may have insulin resistance, you can begin by taking the quiz below. Put a check next to every question for which you answer yes.

Physical Clues

- Are you at least thirty pounds or more overweight?
- Do you gain weight even though you eat small portion sizes and small amounts of food?
- Do you have belly fat, a potbelly, love handles, or weight gain around your waist?
- Is your waist measurement more than forty inches for men or more than thirty-five inches for women?
- Are you of African American, Hispanic, Native American, or Asian ancestry?
- Do you need to urinate frequently?
- Do you experience frequent heartburn or acid reflux?

- Do you have skin tags, which are small, painless skin growths on your chest, neck, breast area, groin area, or underarms?
- Do you have little to no physical activity on most days?

Emotional and Mental Clues

- Do you feel tired after eating, especially in the afternoon, perhaps even feeling the need for a nap?
- Do you experience jitteriness, moodiness, or headaches that go away once you eat?
- Do you experience foggy thinking or difficulty thinking or concentrating at times?
- Do you feel addicted to sodas, candy, and junk food?
- Do you feel you eat out of boredom?
- Do you feel that you have no willpower when it comes to eating or dieting?

Eating and Diet Clues

- Do you crave sweets and carbohydrates, such as pastas and breads?
- Do you crave snacks that are salty and crunchy?
- For breakfast, do you often eat bagels, croissants, or donuts and coffee?
- Do you eat snacks frequently, particularly while watching TV?
- Do you drink sodas or sweetened fruit juice every day?
- Do you drink beer or liquor at least twice a week?
- Do you eat fast foods at least twice per week?

Health or Medical Clues

- Do you have a family history of diabetes, high cholesterol, high blood pressure, heart disease, stroke, or obesity or overweight problems?
- Have you been diagnosed with either type-2 diabetes or hypoglycemia?
- If you are diabetic, do you take a prescription drug to reduce your blood sugar levels?
- Have you been diagnosed with a blood clot in your brain, legs, or lungs?
- Have you been diagnosed with high uric acid or gout?
- Did you grow up around smokers and secondhand smoke?
- If you're a woman, have you been diagnosed with irregular menstrual periods or polycystic ovary syndrome?

If you have marked a check beside fifteen or more questions, then you likely have insulin resistance. Additionally, the more checks you have, the more likely you are to be affected by this condition. To understand additional methods for diagnosing insulin resistance, please see the section below. Today there is not a consensus among the medical community around the best method to diagnose insulin resistance. However, there are a few practical tests that have been used to help determine if someone is insulin resistant. They include the following:

• Waist-circumference measurements: This method is very easy to do. You just use a tape measure to measure your waist circumference. For women, waist measurements of more than thirty-five inches, and for men, more than forty inches, strongly indicate that you have or are at risk for developing insulin resistance.

• Fasting glucose levels: This is a blood test that is simple and can often be done at home. This test measures your blood sugar level after you've been fasting (not eating) for several hours. Normal blood sugar levels are between 80 and 100 mg/dl. Levels that are slightly higher, but not high enough to indicate diabetes, may indicate a condition of insulin resistance.

• Hemoglobin A1C: Hemoglobin A1C, also called HbA1c, evaluates how blood sugar has damaged proteins in your blood. This test will provide a snapshot of your average blood-glucose levels for the past six weeks. The HbA1c test has certain advantages over a fasting glucose test. Sometimes eating a lot of sugary foods the day before a fasting glucose test will throw off the results of the test. Many practitioners prefer this test because the HbA1c shows average blood sugar in recent weeks, whereas a fasting glucose test just shows it based on what a person has eaten recently. Your doctor can order this test for you. To interpret your test results, a normal HbA1c is 4.5 to 5.7 percent; an HbA1c less than 5 percent is ideal. However, many people suffering from insulin resistance or prediabetes have an HbA1c of 5.7 to 6.9 percent, and diabetics have an HbA1c of 7 percent or higher.

Managing Insulin Resistance by Eating "Clean and Balanced" Foods

The bad news is that we cannot change our genetic makeup, and there is no cure for insulin resistance. However, the good news is that insulin resistance can be managed and controlled by eating "clean and balanced foods" and through nutritional supplements that help glucose get inside the cells for energy rather than be stored as fat in the body.

There are two nutritional supplements (alpha-lipoic acid and chromium), which improve insulin function and control your blood sugar levels. Managing insulin resistance not only helps with weight loss, it also prevents numerous other health conditions and diseases. It will take at least two to three months to reestablish normal insulin sensitivity so that your reaction to carbs won't cause your body to store excess fat. However, most people will experience some improvements within two to three weeks after making the adjustments to their diet and taking the nutritional supplements.

What kind of improvements can you expect to experience? Loss of weight, especially around the abdomen, improved energy, and fewer carbohydrate and sugar cravings. Additionally, you will want to get your doctor to monitor your lab results every three to four months, as you will likely have improved blood pressure and blood sugar levels. Lower insulin levels help you lose the unwanted body fat as well as reduce your risk of heart disease and diabetes.

Let's describe what "clean and balanced" foods mean. "Clean" foods are primarily natural, whole, raw, or organic—foods that the body can effectively digest and utilize for energy without leaving excess waste or toxins in the body. "Clean" foods include lean proteins, good carbs, and healthy fats. "Balanced" foods mean that you eat protein every time you eat a carbohydrate. So, if you have carbohydrates, you want to always include protein. It is a very simple but effective method for preventing insulin spikes and aiding the body in burning fat. Why protein every time you eat? Protein counteracts the body's overreaction to carbohydrates, which cause insulin spikes and fat storage. Proteins will also help you feel full longer and thus help prevent overeating and food cravings. Protein will also help you build and maintain muscle mass, and we've learned that muscle naturally burns more calories than fat. Another way to assist with eating "clean and balanced" foods is to use the glycemic index of foods. Foods with a high glycemic response will raise blood glucose dramatically. Foods with a high glycemic response turn into glucose very quickly and therefore cause a rapid rise in insulin levels. We now know that high spikes and rises in insulin levels cause the body to store fat. However, foods that cause a slower glycemic response will not cause insulin levels to rise and are therefore better for people with insulin resistance.

Additionally, there are numerous books and websites available that will list glycemic values for all types of food and beverages. Eating "clean and balanced" foods means eating lean proteins, healthy fats, and more low-glycemic carbs (fruits and veggies), which have little effect on blood sugar and insulin levels and thus prevent the storage of body fat and reduce the risk of diabetes and other health ailments.

Key Factors That Keep Your Hormones Balanced

What causes hormonal imbalance? Too many unhealthy foods, too much stress, and synthetic hormones all cause hormonal imbalances, such as hypothyroidism, leptin resistance, and insulin resistance, which all lead to weight gain. But I will give you the tools to retrain your hormones to perform optimally so you can start losing weight and start feeling balanced, happy, and healthy. Additionally, you may want to work with your doctor to run blood tests to determine if you have any specific hormonal imbalances. The following is a list of ways to keep your hormones balanced.

• Remove excess toxins from your body: The endocrine system, which controls hormone production, is especially sensitive to toxins. When the endocrine system is "disrupted" by toxins, hormone imbalances can occur. The chemicals and toxins in the environment send signals to our bodies that make them produce more or less of our hormones than normal. These toxins, which are "endocrine disruptors," confuse the body, causing it to overreact to their signals, disrupting the normal, healthy functioning of the hormonal system. So, getting rid of toxins is key to balancing your hormones.

• Incorporate healthy, whole foods into your diet: Whole, fresh, and natural foods restore the normal functioning of hormones. These are the foods that trigger your fat-burning hormones and halt your fat storing hormones. When you give your body the foods it was designed to utilize, you support your hormones to do what they're meant to do: make your metabolism work for you, not against you. The foods that help restore your body's metabolism and naturally balance your hormones include legumes (beans); alliums (garlic, onions); berries (blackberries, blueberries, raspberries); veggies, especially dark green, leafy veggies (spinach, kale, collards); nuts and seeds (almonds, pecans, sunflower seeds); and whole grains (oats, barley, quinoa).

• Rebalance your food combinations: This is where eating protein every time you eat a carbohydrate comes into play. The right "balance" among good carbs, healthy fats, and lean proteins allows you to maintain proper blood sugar levels and sustain your energy throughout the day without hunger or cravings. Instead of counting calories, you'll be eating better-quality foods more often throughout the day. I personally get with eating good food more often! The "food" in the Standard American Diet simply doesn't give our hormones what they need to stay balanced. In the next part, I will teach you how to eat "clean and balanced" foods that assist in keeping your hormones balanced.

• Lower your stress levels: You learned earlier that when you are stressed, your body releases a hormone called cortisol, which increases belly fat. Rest, sleep, and relaxation all play a role in lowering the stress in your life. But sometimes you have to "detox" from family and friends who cause you unnecessary stress and strife. People who belittle you and make you feel unworthy should get very little of your time. These people trigger stress and negative emotions in your life. Sometimes they can just say hello, and your stress level increases because you know at the end of that interaction, you will feel low, hurt, or sad. Take steps to minimize the time you spend with these people and find ways to minimize stress in your life. Chronic hormonal imbalances cause you to gain weight and feel moody and fatigued. You will need to detoxify and cleanse your body and your kitchen of the toxic waste that causes you to get fat. You will need to provide your body with healing foods that allow your metabolism to work as a fat-burning machine instead of a fat-storing machine. When your hormones are functioning at their optimal levels, your body is at its peak performance and maintains your healthy, ideal weight.

Speed Up Your Metabolism

Have you tried calorie-counting diets, fat-free diets, small-portions diets, or low-carb diets only to regain every pound you lost while on the diet? Have you tried the weight-loss support meetings and sat next to people who were having success while you looked like you'd been cheating when you really hadn't been? Have you always felt something was wrong or different about your body, especially as you've watched skinny friends eat twice as much as you and not gain a pound? Well, you were probably right. A combination of factors including aging, stress, hormonal changes, and poor food choices all cause a gradual change in metabolism. You are not lazy, and you do not lack willpower or discipline. Your body simply responds differently to food because you have a sluggish metabolism. I know this because I had a sluggish metabolism that slowed in my late thirties. But through studying to become a certified nutritionist specializing in weight management, I began to learn more about my metabolism and its effect on my weight gain. When I first started rapidly gaining weight, I would limit what I ate. I even tried to work out with a trainer but still gained ten to fifteen more pounds. I continued to gain weight despite following the traditional advice of "eat less and exercise more." But my body did not respond to that advice. So, I knew I needed a different and new approach, and I needed it fast. Thank goodness I found it!

If you find it impossible to lose weight and keep it off, even when you follow all the traditional guidance on dieting and exercising, it is very likely that a sluggish metabolism is one of your problems. It is important to understand how your unique body metabolizes food because that determines how food turns into energy or fat in your body. Most diets don't factor in each individual's metabolism. They focus on dietary changes but don't factor in how your individual metabolism is affecting your weight gain. This is why some people have great success with one diet but others get no results from it at all.

If you have a sluggish metabolism, your body won't respond to traditional diets and weight-loss programs. The traditional diet approach of decreasing calories won't work because weight is determined by your body's response to how foods are processed or metabolized within your body. Another problem may be that a lot of your weight loss on diets came not from fat but rather muscle, and you need muscle to keep your metabolic engine running effectively. Muscle cells burn fifty times more calories than fat cells. It is important to lose weight in a manner that ensures you will lose fat and minimize muscle loss, which is what we focus on in the DHEMM System.

How Your Metabolism Affects the Calories You Burn

Metabolism is commonly thought to be a matter of how fast or slowly you burn calories. We often hear people say, "I can't lose weight because I have a slow metabolism." In general, that is true, but metabolism is much more complex. Metabolism represents all the signals and chemical reactions in your body that regulate your weight and the rate at which you burn calories. A number of factors determine how your metabolism processes food and burns calories, including environment, age, food quality, stress levels, genes, and physical activity. Aging, in particular, has a noticeable impact on metabolism, due to changes in hormone balance. Once you understand what controls your metabolism, you will be able to make changes that will automatically turn your body into a fat-burning machine. When you stop focusing on losing weight and instead on restoring your body to its optimal performance level, the weight loss happens effortlessly and automatically. Someone with a high metabolic rate is able to burn calories more efficiently than someone with a slower metabolic rate. Any calories that are not burned get converted to fat. Let's take a look at the three main types of calorie burn that happen throughout your day.

Calorie burn #1: The majority of the calorie burn comes from your basal or resting metabolism, which means you burn calories while you're doing absolutely nothing at all. Yes, 60 to 80 percent of your daily calories are burned up by just doing nothing. Whether it's watching TV, sitting in a meeting at work, or sleeping, you are continuing to burn calories. The reason is that your body is always in a constant state of motion. Your heart is beating, blood is pumping through your veins, and your lungs are breathing. This is another reason I say that exercise is not that important to losing weight. Exercise is important for cardio health, but the calories you burn from exercise don't account for the majority of caloric burn happening throughout the day while doing absolutely nothing (your basal metabolism). The calories you burn during your one hour at the gym are relatively insignificant compared to all the calories you burn during the other twenty-three hours in the day. It's more productive to focus on naturally increasing the rate of your resting metabolism—i.e., your caloric burn throughout the day.

Calorie burn #2: The effect of simply eating and digesting your food accounts for about 10 to 15 percent of the calories you burn each day. Studies have shown that during the eating process, your metabolism increases by as much as 30 percent, and this effect lasts up to three hours after you have finished eating. How much caloric burn occurs depends on the type of food you eat. More caloric burn is used to digest protein (25 calories burned for every 100 calories consumed) than to digest fats and carbohydrates (about 10 to 15 calories burned for every 100 calories consumed). That's why the DHEMM System calls for an appropriate amount of lean, healthy protein.

Calorie burn #3: About 10 to 15 percent of your calorie burn comes from increasing your heart rate, strengthening your muscles, or physical activity, even light physical activity, such as walking up the stairs. In the DHEMM System, we will discuss ways to "get moving" so that you become more physically active throughout each day even if you don't go to the gym or work out.

How to Avoid Slowing Your Metabolism

One of the greatest myths about weight loss is that for some people, it is harder to lose weight because they have a genetically slow metabolism. But scientific research shows that this is simply not true. Your metabolic rate is not fixed for life, and, in fact, it can and will change throughout your lifetime.

Yo-yo dieting will alter your metabolism for the worse and make it more difficult to lose weight in the long term. Some of you who are constantly on diets have probably begun to slow your metabolism unknowingly. Here's how this has happened: When someone goes on a diet, the body notices that it is not getting as much food as it used to or as it needs to, so in order to conserve energy, the body slows its metabolic rate. It also begins storing fat reserves to ensure that it will have enough energy throughout the day. Another problem with endless dieting is that you begin to lose lean muscle mass, which controls your metabolic rate and helps you burn body fat. When the body isn't getting enough food from the diet, it must conserve energy, so the body begins to "eat itself" to get the extra energy it needs.

Thus, in addition to slowing your metabolism, you also may be actually losing muscle mass. Instead of dieting and eating less, you actually want to eat more when you're hungry, which for most people is every three to four hours. Eating every three to four hours signals your body that you have plenty of food and energy to fuel the body throughout the day, causing the body to speed up metabolism to allow the energy to be used most efficiently. Your metabolism will naturally slow as you age. It's true! Your metabolism does slow down with age. Starting at about age twenty-five, the average person's metabolism declines between 5 and 10 percent per decade. So you will have to work harder and be more deliberate about speeding up your metabolism as you age.

If you're like me and over forty, you probably have blamed your weight gain on your slow or sluggish metabolism. Well, you are correct because as you age, your metabolism tends to slow down. Thus, if your resting metabolic rate is, say, 1,200 calories per day at age forty, it will be around 1,140 at age fifty. So after forty, you may have to make dietary or lifestyle changes just to maintain your current weight. Compounding things is the reality that, as we age, life gets more hectic and fast-paced, especially if we work or have children or aging parents. This causes us to eat on the run, which means eating fast foods or less healthy foods because that's all we have time for.

Twelve Ways to Boost Your Metabolism

As I said earlier, you definitely have the ability to speed up or slow down your metabolism. Because everyone's body is different, some of the methods to speed up your metabolism will work extremely well, while others not so well. I know for me, drinking green tea gives me a very noticeable boost in my metabolism because I not only burn fat, I also notice less cellulite as well. Pay close attention to your body and how it responds to each metabolism booster. You will want to incorporate as many metabolism boosters as you can, but it's best to not try them all at the same time so that you can figure out which ones are working well and which ones not so well. Then you can continue with the most effective methods on a consistent, regular basis. Here are twelve easy ways to boost your metabolism to burn more calories:

1. Just stand up: A study by University of Missouri researchers discovered that inactivity (four hours or more) causes a near shutdown of an enzyme that metabolizes fat and cholesterol. This causes you to store more fat as opposed to the body burning fat. If you are going to be sitting for long periods of time, be sure to stand up once in a while and, if possible, simply walk around the room.

2. Eat breakfast: Have a hearty breakfast to rev up your metabolism for the day. Eating a high-protein breakfast wakes up your liver and kicks your metabolism into gear. A high-protein breakfast can increase your metabolic rate by 30 percent for up to twelve hours, which is the calorie-burning equivalent of a three-to five-mile jog. It is important to feed your body every three to four hours and not skip any meals. You especially don't want to skip breakfast. When you skip breakfast, it means your body goes without fuel for about fifteen hours, including the overnight hours. This causes it to automatically store fat over the next twenty-four hours because it thinks it's in starvation mode or a deprived state.

3. Eat more frequently: The goal is to not let more than four hours pass without a meal or snack. Yes, ironically, it is important to eat to lose weight! The number of times you eat is important to keep your metabolism revved up. Every time you eat, you have to burn calories to digest your food, so eating increases your metabolic rate. When more than five hours pass without eating, your body automatically lowers its metabolic rate. In contrast, by eating meals and snacks throughout the day, your body stays at a steady metabolic burn rate that helps you burn calories and fat all day. Remember, we are eating every three or four

hours because eating less will slow your metabolism. It sends a signal to your body that it is starving and deprived, causing the body to respond by slowing the metabolic rate and holding on to existing fat reserves in the body. So, eat more. Yes, you can do that!

4. Don't eat right before going to bed: Eating before bed is a guaranteed way to slow your metabolism and gain weight. The easy solution is to eat dinner and give yourself at least two to three hours after you eat before you go to sleep. You may even want to eat more lightly at dinner and the heaviest at breakfast. Getting more of your energy from your food earlier in the day helps you lose and maintain weight loss because your body can burn fat throughout the entire day. The fat-burning systems in the body slow, rest, and repair at night while you're sleeping.

5. Get as much sleep as you need: One of my favorite ways to boost my metabolism is to get a full eight hours of sleep. When you don't get enough sleep, your energy is low throughout the day. When the body feels tired from a lack of sleep, it seeks to increase energy by consuming food, causing you to crave more sugar, salt, and fats. In late 2004, for example, researchers showed a strong connection between sleep and the ability to lose weight; the more one sleeps, the better the body can regulate the chemicals that control hunger and appetite. One of these hormones is leptin, which is responsible for telling your brain that you are full. When functioning normally, it induces fat burning and reduces fat storage.

6. Get rid of toxins: Toxins can affect your ability to lose weight by slowing down your metabolism and decreasing your ability to burn fat. As toxins circulate in the body, namely the blood, it slows down your resting metabolic rate. In a study in 1971, the University of Nevada's Division of Biochemistry determined that chemical toxins weakened a special coenzyme that the body needs to burn fat by 20 percent. Toxins (pesticides, food additives, herbicides) interfere with the body's fat burning process and make it harder to lose fat.

7. Drink more cold water: German researchers found that if you drink six cups of cold water a day, it can raise resting metabolism by about 50 calories daily, which in a year can help you to shed about five pounds. This is because it takes more work for the body to heat the water to your body temperature. This is a small thing that can help you lose weight with very little effort. The German researchers also suggest that for up to 90 minutes after drinking cold water, you will keep your metabolism boosted by as much as 24 percent over your average metabolic rate.

8. Drink caffeinated coffee or tea: Caffeine is a central nervous system stimulant and can speed up your metabolism by 5 to 8 percent, which helps to burn about 100 to 175 calories a day. This does not mean you should overdo it and drink several cups of coffee. Having one cup of coffee is sufficient, but too many cups of coffee can have adverse side effects. Additionally, green tea, my favorite metabolism booster, is found to provide many health benefits to the body.

9. Build lean muscle: As you get older, you will want to maintain as much muscle mass as possible. If you lose muscle mass, your metabolic rate will begin to slow, and you'll burn fewer calories. In fact, one pound of fat burns about two calories

a day to maintain itself, whereas one pound of lean muscle mass burns thirty to fifty calories a day to maintain itself. So just by maintaining more muscle mass, you will burn more calories throughout the day and keep your metabolism revved up. Putting on just five to ten pounds of lean muscle mass will speed up your resting metabolism so you will burn more calories even when you're resting.

10. Eat more fiber: Research shows that fiber can increase your fat burning by as much as 30 percent. Aim for about 30 grams per day, through either fiber-rich foods or fiber supplements. In fact, there's even a diet whose focus is solely on increasing daily fiber intake as a method to lose weight.

11. Get moving: Physical activity of any kind speeds up metabolism, and aerobic exercise gives it a significant boost. Also, the higher the intensity of the aerobic exercise, the more it will help your metabolism remain elevated for an extended period of time, so that you continue to burn calories even after you have stopped exercising.

12. Spice it up: One study showed that hot or spicy peppers (chili or cayenne peppers) caused a temporary metabolism boost of about 23 percent. Some people have even purchased cayenne pepper capsules to supplement spicy pepper into their diet daily just to boost their metabolism.

Foods That Speed Up Metabolism

Certain foods are especially effective in speeding up metabolism. They do so in one of three ways: by helping to maintain hormonal balance; by reducing insulin levels, which control fat storage; and by increasing muscle mass (via protein), as muscle burns more calories than fat. These "magic" foods include:

• Whey or rice protein powder: Whey protein, which comes from cow's milk, is a complete high-quality protein that speeds up metabolism. If you are a vegetarian, you can use rice protein to accomplish the same thing.

• Nuts and seeds: Nuts and seeds provide healthy fats that raise the body's metabolism.

• Green tea: Studies have shown that green tea is one of the best metabolism boosters you can drink.

• Beans: Beans are loaded with fiber, which helps you feel full longer, preventing cravings and binges.

• Berries: Berries are packed with antioxidants and keep your metabolism going strong. Eat them fresh or frozen.

• Cayenne pepper: Cayenne pepper is known as a fat burner because it fires up your metabolism. It heats up the body, and the body burns calories when it cools itself down.

• Green smoothies: A blend of green leafy vegetables, fruits, and water.

• Vegetables: Vegetables contain fiber, vitamins, and many essential nutrients that help keep metabolism elevated.

• Whole grain cereals: Cereals such as oatmeal boost the metabolism by keeping insulin levels low after you eat. If you secrete too much insulin, it results in the storage of body fat, which slows down your metabolism.

• Lean beef, pork, chicken, and turkey: These are all good sources of lean protein. The more protein you eat, the harder your body has to work to digest it, resulting in more calories burned during the eating process.

• Salmon, tuna, and sardines: These fish contain omega-3 fatty acids. French researchers found that men who replaced 6 grams of fat in their diets with 6 grams of fish oil (omega-3 fatty acids) were able to boost their metabolisms and lose an average of two pounds in just twelve weeks. Wild Pacific salmon, in particular, is loaded with omega-3 fats and is a very healthy fish.

Once you begin to boost your metabolism, the weight will come off andstay off permanently. Not only that, but your health will improve as well. You can learn how your body works and how to speed up your metabolism so you burn more calories and fat throughout each day. You'll learn how to get energy from your foods to sustain you all day and keep your metabolism revved up. Weight-related health problems will diminish and, in some cases, even disappear.

Eat Foods That Make You Thin

When you eat foods that are primarily natural, whole, raw, or organic, your body can more effectively deal with digesting and utilizing these foods. Healthy foods are recognizable by the body and can be broken down, whereas unnatural foods and ingredients cannot be broken down and will actually cause weight gain, premature aging, and other ailments. The healthiest foods are those that are the easiest for the body to digest—they are effectively broken down and utilized and leave little waste or toxins in the body. In this section, we will discuss the following:

- The three foundation foods
- Fiber
- Beverages
- Nutritional supplements

You have probably heard a lot about the need to eat "whole foods." What are whole foods? Whole foods are foods that are fresh and unprocessed and remain almost exactly in the form that they were found in nature. Whole foods include beans, vegetables, whole grains, fruits, nuts, and seeds. As we stated earlier, the quicker your body is able to break down and digest food, the less waste matter it leaves behind that eventually turns into fat cells in the body. Additionally, the longer it takes the body to break down food to digest it, the longer you'll feel full and satisfied throughout the day.

You also hear a lot about organic foods, which are free from chemical preservatives, additives, hormones, pesticides, and antibiotics. Fresh organic foods are far less toxic than highly processed and packaged/frozen foods. Organic foods support good health and help you maintain your ideal weight as well as detoxify the body. Fresh organic fruits, vegetables, whole grains, and meats are best for you. Frozen fruits and vegetables retain many vitamins and often don't contain as many preservatives as packaged and canned foods, but they lack vital enzymes needed for the body to digest them properly. Frozen dinners and canned, boxed, and instant foods are the least healthy options because they often contain sugar, salt, preservatives, and unhealthy fats.

The Three Foundation Foods for Healthy Eating

The three foundation foods for the DHEMM System are lean proteins, good carbohydrates (carbs), and healthy fats. What you eat is the most important factor in losing weight. You can do all the exercising you want, but if you do not feed your body the necessary foods with the right nutrients, then you will hinder your progress toward your weight-loss goals. Knowing what to eat is essential to staying slim. Eating a healthy, well-balanced meal with lean proteins, good carbohydrates, and healthy fats will help you lose weight and keep it off. What I have learned from counseling my clients is that most people don't know the differences between proteins, carbohydrates, and fats. For instance, many people don't know that fruits and vegetables are carbohydrates. It's important for you to start to think of all foods as either proteins, carbs, or fats. This information is critical to managing your weight long term because each type of food has different hormonal impacts affecting weight gain.

• Lean proteins: One of the most effective nutrients for speeding up metabolism and building muscle in he body is protein. Protein boosts the caloric burn while it is being digested and helps to build muscle that also helps burn calories. Examples of lean proteins include eggs, fish, lean poultry, or lean beef (preferably organic and grass-fed or free-range meat).

• Good carbs: Carbohydrates, particularly those found in their natural form, contain most of the essential nutrients that keep you healthy, give you energy, and turn up your metabolism. Examples include fruit, vegetables, whole grains, beans, nuts, and seeds.

• Healthy fats: Healthy fats are the good fats—those that have omega-3 fatty acids that help speed up your metabolism and help your body burn fat more quickly. Examples include fish oil; extra-virgin olive oil; cold pressed plant oils, such as grape seed oil and sesame oil; nuts and seeds; and coconut.

Every one of your body parts, including your blood, skin, organs, enzymes, and muscles, requires protein. High-protein foods are extremely effective for speeding up metabolism naturally. As I explained earlier, the body uses more calories to digest protein than it does to digest carbs or fat. According to a 2006 Journal of Clinical Nutrition study, consuming nearly a third of your daily calories as lean protein will increase your metabolism not only during the day, but also when you're sleeping. Additionally, consuming enough protein helps you preserve lean muscle mass, and the more lean muscle you have, the more calories you burn, even at rest. Eating protein balances your blood-sugar levels so you don't get spikes in energy. It also helps the liver stay metabolically active, especially if you eat it at breakfast, as this helps provide a stable base for energy, mood, and blood sugar throughout the day and evening. For this reason, eating protein at breakfast will help you if you tend to crash in the afternoon. When choosing protein, you must understand that not all proteins are created equal. You want to be sure you're eating high-quality, lean proteins that have the essential amino acids required to grow, build, and maintain muscle mass, enabling your body to burn more calories throughout the day.

Now that we know that protein can help you lose those unwanted pounds, it's important to eat the right amount and the right kind of proteins to get the health benefits. An average person requires about 50 to 70 grams of protein each day. Five to eight servings of lean protein foods should meet this need. Although a detailed list of lean protein options is provided in next part, here are some guidelines for selecting good sources of lean protein.

- Fish

Fish is one of the healthiest sources of lean protein because it is lower in saturated fat than beef or poultry. Good fish choices include wild salmon, tuna, and sardines. Salmon is extremely healthy and is a good food to eat if you want to shed excess weight. It has an abundance of healthy omega-3 fats, which encourage fat burning. If you have a choice of salmon, always pick the wild-caught kind instead of the cheaper farmed salmon. The most abundant source of wild salmon is found in Alaska, but Canada, California, and a few other states offer it as well. Although both wild and farmed salmon have equivalent levels of omega-3s, compared to wild salmon, farmed salmon is higher in toxins and other chemicals. Wild salmon also is richer in astaxanthin, a very potent antioxidant, anti-inflammatory nutrient popular in the anti-aging industry. Most farmed salmon is fed synthetic astaxanthin, which is inferior to the natural form of this nutrient. Many chefs also use wild salmon because of its superior flavor and texture. Try to eat salmon at least twice a week.

- Poultry

Boneless, skinless chicken or turkey breast meat is ideal. Because the skin is loaded with saturated fat, be sure to remove it before cooking. I know the skin adds flavor, but it also adds fat and calories. When choosing poultry, choose white-meat turkey and chicken as often as possible; it is lower in calories than dark meat. The best ways to prepare poultry are roasting, grilling, or baking. Avoid frying because that adds calories.

- Beef

Just because you're watching your fat and calorie intake doesn't mean you have to give up beef altogether. If you buy ground beef, get the kind that is 90 percent lean or higher. The label on the package should read "lean" or "extra lean." Choose "choice" or "select" sirloin, flank, top round, London broil, or chuck, which are usually leaner cuts of meat. Avoid meats that say "prime"—these are flavorful but a bit more fatty. In general, you don't want to eat too much red meat on a weekly basis; however, if you do choose to eat red meats, at least buy meat from grass-fed rather than grain-fed animals. The ranchers who run feedlots typically feed grain to their livestock because it's cheaper and makes their animals fatter and heavier, but the meat from these animals is less nutritious than that from grass-fed animals. Furthermore, grain-fed cattle often have synthetic hormones, antibiotics, and other additives that are passed down to us when we eat their meat. In general, meat from grass-fed animals is lower in fat, cholesterol, and calories. Of course, most supermarket meats are from grain fed animals, so you may have to go to a Whole Foods or natural grocery store to find the healthier kind. If you are buying poultry or eggs, you'll also want to look for the meat (and eggs) of free-range rather than grain-fed animals.

The following health benefits, according to Jo Robinson, author of Why Grass-fed Is Best, are derived from eating meats from grass-fed as opposed to grain-fed cattle:

• A 6-ounce steak from a grass-fed steer has almost 100 fewer calories than one from a grain-fed animal.

• Meat from grass-fed animals has half the saturated fat of that from grain-fed animals.

• Meat from grass-fed animals has two to six times more omega-3 fats (healthy fats) than that from grain-fed animals.

• Beans

Beans, lentils, and peas are also good lean protein sources and have the added benefit of being high in fiber. The protein and fiber content of beans, peas, and lentils will help you feel full longer and prevent overeating. You could easily add them to salads, chili, or soups. Beans and legumes are also carbohydrates but are not as quickly digested as most other carbohydrates, so they function more like high-protein food sources.

• Eggs

Eggs received bad press for many years due to cholesterol concerns, but eggs can be included in any healthy diet. If you do have cholesterol concerns, just avoid the yolks, which contain all of the fat and cholesterol. Egg whites are a good high-protein, low-cholesterol choice. An omelet made from one yolk and two egg whites hardly tastes any different from one made from two entire eggs—and it is lower in fat and cholesterol. As I'll discuss in the next section, I am not a fan of dairy products. However, if you do choose to eat or drink dairy products, they should be fat free or low-fat with no added sugar. This makes unsweetened low-fat or nonfat yogurt or cottage cheese a good protein food source.

• Good Carbs

Carbohydrates constitute the biggest group of foods we eat. Those found in their natural form contain most of the essential nutrients that give us energy and fuel our body throughout the day. Foods like sugar, white breads, and white pasta have given carbs a bad rap. But the world of carbs is actually much broader than this. Carbohydrates supply vitamins and minerals, particularly thiamin, niacin, and the powerful antioxidant vitamin E. They are also important sources of fiber, which is an essential nutrient for controlling appetite and making you feel full longer. In short, your body needs carbohydrates not only for energy but also to make serotonin, an important brain chemical that tells you when you are full and no longer hungry.

Unfortunately, most of the carbs that Americans eat are the "bad carbs" found in candy, sweets, junk foods, sodas, fruit juice, sugary cereals, breads, rice, and pasta. The problem with "bad carbs" is that they don't metabolize in our bodies properly, causing insulin spikes, which eventually lead to insulin resistance, causing fat storage in the body. But did you know fruits and vegetables are also carbohydrates? Nuts, seeds, beans, and whole grains are also carbs. These are all "good" carbs, and if you want to be thin and healthy, you must include these "good" carbs in your diet. The "good" carbs contain very important ingredients necessary for optimal health and should be a big part of your diet. These include:

- Nuts and seeds
- Whole grains
- Beans
- Fruits
- Vegetables

Nuts and seeds. If you are trying to lose weight, add nuts and seeds to your diet. Nuts and seeds provide energy and build stamina because they are such a powerhouse of nutrients. Studies have shown that some nuts and seeds in your diet actually aids in appetite suppression and weight loss. You don't want to eat an entire bag of nuts and seeds because they are calorie-rich, so don't overeat. Organic, raw nuts and seeds are a better nutritional choice than roasted nuts, which typically are heavy with added oils and salt. A few choices of nuts and seeds include almonds, Brazil nuts, pine nuts, walnuts, macadamia nuts, sesame seeds, and sunflower seeds. Whole grains. Although whole grains have been recommended because they are high in fiber and rich in vitamin E and B complex, a recent Harvard study published in the Journal of Clinical Nutrition showed that whole grains also help you lose weight and prevent weight gain. The Harvard research concluded that women who eat the most whole grains have a 49 percent lower risk of gaining weight and a much lower risk of developing heart disease and diabetes. This research proved that women can lose more weight and maintain their weight loss better than those who eat a lesser amount of whole grains. When you look for whole grains, search for the least processed, 100 percent whole grain cereals, breads, and pasta. As an example, when you eat oatmeal (a whole grain source), be sure it is rolled oats or oat flakes rather than the instant variety of oatmeals that have added sugar.

Healthy whole grain options include barley, oats, bulgur, corn, millet, quinoa, brown rice, whole wheat, and buckwheat.

Beans: There are many different kinds of beans, including black beans, lentils, red kidney beans, pinto beans, split peas, chickpeas (garbanzo beans), lima beans, and butter beans. If eating beans gives you gas, you can significantly reduce that problem by soaking the beans overnight and pouring out the soaked water before cooking. Fruits. Fruits provide tremendous health benefits to our bodies by supplying vital amino acids, minerals, and vitamins. Fruit breaks down faster than any other food in our system, leaving us fueled and energized; and because it is a highly cleansing food, it leaves no toxic residue in the body. In fact, fruit dissolves toxic substances and cleanses our tissues, even eliminating old toxic residue in our bodies. In short, fruit is the most life-enhancing food you can eat. Fruits are carbohydrates that are high in fiber and water. Some healthy fruits include blueberries, apples, grapefruit, kiwi, cantaloupe, papaya, blackberries, cherries, and grapes.

Vegetables: In order to be lean, strong, and healthy, you must eat vegetables every day. Studies have shown that those who eat a large variety of vegetables have the least amount of body fat. Green leafy vegetables are especially important because they are low in calories, rich in nutrients, and very high in fiber. This category of vegetables includes kale, spinach, collards, turnip greens, mustard greens, and beet greens. Other vegetables include asparagus, broccoli, carrots, eggplant, celery, peppers, cabbage, cauliflower, Brussels sprouts, and radishes. If you are trying to lose weight, you should limit your intake of starchy vegetables, such as potatoes and corn, as they are higher in calories. Starchy vegetables are also high on the glycemic index, which means they get absorbed into the bloodstream rapidly and cause a surge in insulin levels, leading to excess fat storage in the body.

When you reach your desired weight and your weight becomes more stable, you can begin to add the more starchy vegetables to your meals. You should eat as many fruits and vegetables as possible. A great way to minimize weight gain is to make sure you eat fresh, high-quality, ideally organic fruits and vegetables. One simple way to boost your fruit and vegetable intake is to juice them or drink a green drink daily. A green drink, which we'll discuss later in this section, gives you the equivalent of about five servings of vegetables in one drink. I recommend this at least once a day in the morning. I strongly believe that eating vegetables raw, juicing vegetables, or consuming green drinks is key to being slim, radiant, healthy, and energetic.

Buy organic fruits and veggies whenever possible. Certain fruits and veggies, such as strawberries, peaches, pears, nectarines, cherries, grapes, apples, bell peppers, carrots, celery, and greens (such as kale and lettuce), are covered with toxic pesticides and agricultural chemicals. Always look to buy organic when it comes to these fruits and veggies. For other types, such as those with an inedible skin, it is not as critical to buy organic. These include avocados, bananas, papayas, pineapples, watermelon, kiwis, mangoes, onions, sweet corn, and sweet peas. Also lower in pesticides are asparagus, cabbage, and eggplant. If you can't afford organic fruits and vegetables, wash off the pesticides and waxes as best you can. Waxes are pretty difficult to remove; in fact, they usually can't be removed by simply washing them. You need to purchase special cleansers from health food stores. Be sure to rinse the produce after you scrub off the wax. You can also reduce the toxic content of fruits and vegetables by soaking and scrubbing them in a tub of 10 percent white vinegar and then washing them off with water.

- Healthy Fats

Most people believe that low-fat diets are the best way to lose weight, but this is not true. Healthy fats, such as fish oils and coconut oil, not only encourage weight loss but also help you heal many illnesses and ailments. Healthy fats are needed to produce hormones in the body and provide the body with essential fatty acids. However, you should avoid eating large amounts of any fatty foods, as they are high in calories and will cause you to gain weight. There are essentially three different kinds of fat: healthy fats, bad fats, and ugly fats. I will discuss the good ones here and educate you about the bad and ugly ones in the next section. The healthy fats are the unsaturated fats, and they should be included in your diet every day. The best sources of healthy, unsaturated fats are fish, flax oil, fish oil, hemp oil, corn oil, safflower oil, walnuts, sunflower seeds, and pumpkin seeds. An easy way to transition healthy oils into your diet is to use flax oil as a salad dressing, use olive oil for cooking, and take fish oil supplements for added benefit.

You may often hear about a certain type of healthy fat, called omega-3 fatty acids, which are essential unsaturated fats. Healthy omega-3 fats are in nuts and seeds, flaxseeds, pumpkin seeds, walnuts, hazelnuts, pistachios, almonds, Brazil nuts, cashews, and different types of wild fish, including wild salmon, herring, and sardines. Nuts and seeds are a great healthy snack packed with protein, fiber, and healthy fats. However, if you are overweight and want to maximize your weight loss, you should limit your intake of nuts and seeds to one serving (one ounce) per day because they are so calorie-rich. But you should not exclude these healthy fats completely from your diet. As long as you don't overeat nuts and seeds, consuming them, preferably raw, has been found to promote weight loss and appetite suppression, not weight gain. To understand how many nuts is appropriate for a snack, just think "a handful."

A handful (or what you hold in your palm) is generally one ounce. Fill up an empty Altoids box with nuts so you have your handy snack with you at all times. If you prefer to count them out, it would be about forty pistachios, twenty almonds, twenty pecan halves, eighteen macadamia nuts, eighteen cashews, or fifteen walnut halves. You don't want to sit in front of the TV and eat an entire bag of nuts while watching your favorite television show. Healthy eating means avoiding excessive calories and not eating for recreation. Be disciplined about how you snack and be sure to not eat out of boredom.

Nuts are also richer in minerals and vitamins than animal proteins, and nut protein is easily assimilated and does not create uric acid. Raw nuts and seeds are a better nutritional choice than roasted nuts, which are usually loaded with added oil and salt. Roasted nuts also lose their freshness more quickly. If you prefer dry-roasted nuts, dry roast your own nuts gently at a low oven temperature, around 150°F, for about ten to fifteen minutes.

Eating Fiber to Lose Weight

If you are trying to lose weight, fiber is known as a miracle nutrient that helps to regulate blood sugar, control hunger, and increase the feeling of fullness (satiety), which will help you lose and maintain your ideal weight for a lifetime. What is fiber? Fiber is the indigestible part of fruits, seeds, vegetables, whole grains, and other edible plants. Processed foods and refined sugars in our diet have taken the place of fiber-rich fruits and vegetables, leaving us vulnerable to poor health and weight gain. However, eating about 30 grams of fiber per day will help you lose weight, prevent disease, and achieve optimum health. Fiber-rich foods make you feel full, but they are not high-calorie foods, meaning you get to eat a lot of food without consuming a lot of calories. Fiber is a natural appetite suppressant; it curbs your appetite so that you can more easily reduce your caloric intake. Fiber will also improve your digestion and help you maintain bowel regularity.

According to Brenda Watson, author of The Fiber35 Diet: Nature's Weight Loss Secret, for every gram of fiber you eat, you can potentially eliminate seven calories. This means that if you consume 35 grams of fiber daily, you will burn 245 extra calories a day. There are two basic types of fiber—soluble and insoluble. Soluble fiber dissolves and breaks down in water, forming a thick gel. Some food sources of soluble fiber include apples, oranges, peaches, nuts, barley, beets, carrots, cranberries, lentils, oats, bran, and peas. Soluble fiber slows the absorption of food after meals and thus helps regulate blood sugar and insulin levels, reducing fat storage in the body. It also removes unwanted toxins, lowers cholesterol, and reduces the risk of heart disease and gallstones. Insoluble fiber (also known as roughage) does not dissolve in water or break down in your digestive system. Insoluble fiber passes through the gastrointestinal tract almost intact. Some food sources of insoluble fiber include green leafy vegetables, seeds and nuts, fruit skins, potato skins, vegetable skins, wheat bran, and whole grains. Insoluble fiber not only promotes weight loss and relieves constipation, but it also assists in the removal of cancer-causing substances from the colon wall. It helps to prevent the formation of gallstones by binding with bile acids and removing cholesterol before stones can form, thus they are especially beneficial to people with diabetes or colon cancer.

You will want to consume both soluble and insoluble fiber because each type provides benefits to the body. Many health organizations recommend that people consume 20 to 35 grams of fiber per day, not to exceed 50 grams. To support weight-loss efforts and improve colon and digestive health, I recommend a fiber intake of a minimum of 30 grams per day. The average American consumes only 10 to 15 grams of fiber daily. If you're increasing your fiber intake, it is important to drink plenty of water to avoid constipation. A good rule of thumb is to drink half your body weight in ounces of water daily. To determine how much this is, just divide your body weight (in pounds) by two and drink that number of ounces of water per day. As an example, if you weigh 140 pounds, then you want to drink 70 ounces (about nine 8-oz glasses) of water daily.

The best way to get more fiber in your diet is through foods high in fiber. A few high-fiber food choices are:

- 1 cup bran cereal (20g)
- 1 cup cooked black beans (14g)
- 1 cup red cooked lentil beans (13g)
- 1 cup cooked kidney beans (12g)
- 1 medium avocado (12g)
- 1 cup oats (12g)
- 1 cup cooked peas (9g)
- 1 cup cooked lima beans (9g)
- 1 cup brown rice (8g)
- 1 cup cooked kale (7g)
- 3 tablespoons flaxseeds (7g)

- 1 cup raspberries (6g)
- 1/2 cup sunflower seeds (6g)
- 1 medium apple (5g)
- 1 medium pear (5g)
- 1 cup cooked broccoli (5g)
- 1 cup cooked carrots (5g)
- 1 medium baked potato or sweet potato (5g)
- 1 cup blueberries (4g)
- 1 cup strawberries (4g)
- 1 medium banana (4g)
- 1 ounce almonds (4g)
- 1 cup cooked spinach (4g)
- 3 cups air-popped popcorn (4g)
- 1 ounce walnuts or pistachios (3g)

If you don't get enough fiber in your diet, you might want to try supplements. I have personally used psyllium but had a lot of trouble with gas, bloating, and constipation. I recommend acacia, flax, or oat fibers as a better alternative for a fiber supplement. In addition to fiber supplements, you can eat fiber bars or drink fiber shakes to increase your daily fiber intake.

- Beverages That Help You Stay Slim and Healthy

Now we want to focus on the best drinks and beverages that help us lose weight and stay healthy. The best choices are the following:

- Water
- Green smoothies
- Green tea
- Fresh-squeezed juices
- Coconut water
- Non-dairy milk

Water: The most important thing to drink for weight loss and good health is water! On average, your body is 60 to 70 percent water, with about two-thirds of it in your cells and the rest in your blood and body fluids. Therefore, water is essential to a healthy, functioning body. Water flushes out toxins and supports every metabolic process in the body, carrying toxins and waste away from cells to the kidneys to be removed from the body. The funny thing is that drinking too little water every day actually causes your body to retain water. The kidneys require an adequate amount of water to flush waste from the body. When the body is lacking water, the kidneys begin to hoard water and the lymphatic system becomes sluggish. You have to keep your body well hydrated. You want to drink plenty of water throughout the day. Drink at least half your body weight in ounces every day. To determine if you are getting enough water and are well hydrated, look at your urine. If it is yellow, you're dehydrated and need to drink more water. The goal is to get your urine as clear in color as possible.

Water can also help minimize cravings. At times, you may feel as though you are craving certain foods, but in actuality, you are just dehydrated. So, anytime you crave sweets, drink some water first. You may find that the craving goes away after drinking water. As it relates to detoxification, an even better type of water is alkaline water. At a minimum, you should drink spring or filtered water (at least half your body weight in ounces), but for truly beautiful, hydrated skin, try alkaline water. Alkaline water detoxifies the body, leaving the skin looking smoother and more elastic and restoring it to a more youthful state. Alkaline water is known for hydrating the skin and keeping the inner body balanced and clean. If you decide to try alkaline water, start out with just a little at first to avoid strong detox symptoms.

Green tea: Green tea has tremendous health benefits. It is one of the few caffeinated drinks that I strongly recommend. In fact, it is an integral part of the DHEMM System. Green tea is particularly helpful with reducing body fat and weight, stimulating digestion, and preventing high blood pressure. It has been shown to be twenty times more effective in slowing the aging process than vitamin E because of its strong antioxidant capacity. The vitamin C content of green tea is four times higher than that of lemon juice. There are many wonderful benefits of drinking green tea, but as far as weight loss goes, it simply helps the body burn fat faster and more efficiently.

Green tea is better than black tea or coffee because its caffeine works in a different way. Green tea makes the body's own energy use more efficient, thereby improving your vitality and stamina without your having to experience the up-and-down effect typically experienced with caffeine. This is due to the large amounts of tannins in green tea that ensure that the caffeine is taken to the brain in only small amounts, which harmonizes the energies in the body.

Green tea is very high in antioxidants, but since it does contain caffeine, don't drink it too late in the day or it can interfere with sleep. I strongly recommend that you enjoy green tea (either hot or iced tea) in the morning and for lunch. For detoxification purposes, I recommend one to two cups a day. If you prefer, you may take one green tea capsule two to three times a day instead. My favorite brand is Wu-Long Chinese Slimming Tea.

Just a quick aside about caffeine: About half the research shows caffeine from coffee and tea to be beneficial, and about half suggests it has detrimental effects on the body. I'm with the half that says it can be beneficial and can improve the fat-burning process. Thus, I recommend drinking some caffeine drinks like green tea or coffee in moderation as a part of the DHEMM System.

Fresh-squeezed juices: Fresh-squeezed juices, as opposed to store-bought juices that have additives and sugar, are also very important to your health. Fresh fruits and vegetables are extremely high in enzymes. Enzymes are actually organic catalysts that increase the rate at which food is broken down and absorbed by the body. However, these enzymes are destroyed during cooking and processing, as well as in bottled and packaged juices, so try to eat them fresh or juice them whenever possible. Fresh juice contains living digestive enzymes that are important in breaking down foods in the digestive tract. This preserves your body's own digestive enzymes, giving your digestive system a much-needed rest so that it can repair, recuperate, and rejuvenate. Additionally, fresh juices are rich in phytonutrients, which are important plant-derived nutrients that contain antioxidants that slow the aging process.

Coconut water: Water or juice from young coconuts is a super-hydrating kind of water that is not only delicious but also rich in minerals, especially potassium. It has almost twice as much potassium as a banana. Drinking it is an excellent way to replace electrolytes after a heavy workout or simply to hydrate the body on a hot day. Many athletes and runners drink coconut water instead of sports drinks like Gatorade. It is fat-and cholesterol-free and low in calories, with positive effects on circulation, body temperature, heart function, and blood pressure.

Coconut water is simply an outstanding beverage for so many reasons. It is my personal favorite these days. In tropical regions, it has been used for centuries as a health and beauty aid because it naturally hydrates the skin. It has a natural balance of sodium, potassium, calcium, and magnesium, making it a healthy drink for hydrating and replacing electrolytes in the body. It is low in calories and has been shown to have antiviral and antifungal properties. The brands I enjoy the most are Vita Coco and O.N.E. Coconut Water.

Non-dairy milk: As I'll discuss in the next section, there are many reasons to give up cow's milk (dairy), but milk is an important part of a healthy diet. The goal should be to drink healthier milk options. Dairy products made from the milk of goats and sheep are better than those made from cow's milk, particularly if they are raw. The natural enzymes in goat's milk are far closer to those in humans, so we're able to digest goat's milk significantly better. Sheep's milk is the next best choice. There are also non-dairy milk options, such as almond, rice, hemp, or soy milk (all unsweetened). If you still decide to consume products made with cow's milk, buy organic and fat free or low-fat brands because they are more nutritious.

Nutritional Supplements

No matter how well we eat, it is likely that there will be some nutrients we just don't get quite enough of. Therefore, we should consume high-quality nutritional supplements. Supplements help you maintain your weight, achieve optimal health, fight disease, and slow the aging process. As it relates to weight loss, I recommend nutritional supplements that will help you lose body fat, preserve muscle mass, and regulate levels of blood sugar and insulin, which are critical for maintaining a healthy, slim body. Scientific research has proven that various supplements can help the body better metabolize fats, reduce the inflammation coming from fat cells, and fill in nutritional gaps and deficiencies. The supplements I recommend go beyond the typical multivitamins. These recommended supplements, combined with dietary changes, are your secret weapons against excess fat in the body. Supplements are a part of the DHEMM System for maintaining good health as you age.

What I discuss in this section is a general overview of supplements to provide basic knowledge that you can then take to your physician and local health food store to get specifics on dosage or on how much of a given supplement to take given your current health. Where possible, I will provide my suggestions, but as always, consult your doctor prior to starting any new diet, supplement, or exercise regimen. These supplements can help support detoxification, strengthen the immune system, balance hormones, protect against degenerative diseases, and promote weight loss. Supplements recommended in the DHEMM System include the following:

- Green drinks
- Fiber
- Fish oil (omega-3 fatty acids)
- Protein drinks
- Antioxidants
- Probiotics
- Vitamin C
- Digestive enzymes
- Nutritional supplements
- Alpha-lipoic acid or R-lipoic acid (for those who are insulin-resistant only)
- Chromium (for those who are insulin-resistant only)

Please note that these supplements do not have to be taken individually. Many are found in multivitamins or in green drinks. As an example, a product called Green Vibrance provides probiotics, digestive enzymes, antioxidants, and fiber. Additionally, the protein drink I use by Rainbow Light, Acai Berry Blast Protein Energizer, contains sufficient quantities of protein, digestives enzymes, antioxidants, and fiber.

Green drinks: One of the most important supplements I include in the DHEMM System is nicknamed the "green drink" because it is derived primarily from green leafy vegetables, the same greens that feed some of the strongest, biggest animals on the planet, such as cows, horses, and oxen. Green drinks help you detoxify and cleanse your system, lose weight, have more energy, and make the body more alkaline. When you drink them, the nutrients in them get to the cells very quickly and give the body a real boost.

The green drink I recommend is a high-density nutrient powder (Vitamineral Green) primarily composed of greens including kale, spinach, alfalfa, barley grass, wheatgrass, broccoli, and many others. These greens are harvested at their peak, dried, and lightly processed into powders. This innovative process preserves most of their vitamins, minerals, nutrients, phytochemicals, and enzymes. You simply mix a scoop of the green powder with water or juice, drink it down, and voilà! You just drank five servings of fruits and veggies! I can get extremely busy some days and can't trust that I will eat enough fruits and veggies, so this ensures that I'm covered even before I leave home. When I travel, I have individual packets of my green drink to carry with me on the road. I never leave home without my green drink! Another great green drink option is made by Green Vibrance; it also contains green leafy vegetables and provides probiotics, digestive enzymes, and antioxidants. If you want to begin by adding only one recommended nutritional supplement into your diet, it should be the green drink.

Fiber: In the DHEMM System, I recommend that you get at least 30 grams of fiber per day. If you are unable to get 30 grams a day of fiber from your food, there are a few convenient supplement options.

• Chewable fiber wafers: Try eating a couple of acacia-based chewable fiber wafers. Ask your local health food store for help in finding these.

• Clear fiber powder: Clear, tasteless, zero-calorie acacia fiber can be sprinkled on your food to enhance the fiber content without altering the taste of your meals. One of my favorite brands is called Fiber35 Diet Sprinkle Fiber by Fiber35 Diet.

• Shakes: Look for shakes that have at least 10 grams of fiber (from acacia) per serving and a decent amount of whey protein (around 20 grams) from a rich source, as well as a variety of important vitamins, minerals, and enzymes to improve digestion. Avoid shakes that contain artificial sugar substitutes. A natural sweetener like stevia is best.

• Bars: Look for high-fiber bars that contain about 10 grams of fiber (6 soluble, 4 insoluble) from oat bran, gum acacia, and milled flaxseed, and 10 grams of protein from whey protein concentrate. Look for a bar that is sweetened with dates, raisins, and stevia or agave syrup.

Fish oil (Omega-3 Fatty Acids): Supplementing your diet with fish oil helps eliminate excess fat while also rejuvenating the cells in the body. Taking a good-quality fish oil supplement will provide you with the necessary omega-3 fatty acids you need to burn stored fat and maintain optimum health. A high-quality fish oil supplement supplies a concentrated amount of the two important omega-3 fatty acids: EPA and DHA. Fish oil/cod liver oil (ultra-refined EPA/DHA concentrates) is considered a wonder drug for its amazing health benefits. Many people take liquid fish oil instead of capsules, particularly if they want a higher dosage of EPA and DHA. If you do use liquid fish oil, always keep it in the refrigerator to prevent oxidation and to preserve its taste. One of my favorite brands is made by Carlson Labs—I like its quality and light lemon taste.

Protein drinks: One quick and easy way to ensure you get more protein in your diet is to take a protein powder supplement. Supplementing protein in your diet should help you stay slim, maintain muscle mass, and slow aging. Whey protein (cow's milk) is a high-quality, complete protein source. However, a non-dairy rice protein will also provide benefits for those who want to stay away from dairy. Protein is essential for weight loss because your body uses more energy to digest protein than other foods so it helps you burn more calories. It also helps to slow down the absorption of glucose in the bloodstream, reducing insulin levels, making it easier for the body to burn fat, and decrease hunger between meals. Protein also preserves lean muscle tissue, and by maintaining muscle mass in the body, you keep your metabolism higher, which will naturally burn more calories.

Antioxidants: Taking an antioxidant supplement will help your body repair cellular damage. Antioxidants work to sweep up dangerous free radicals that can interfere with cellular function. Two more power hitters in the antioxidants are L-carnitine and coenzyme Q10. L-carnitine is an amino acid that ushers fats through the cells to the mitochondria where they can be used for fuel. The food with the highest concentration of L-carnitine is avocado. The mitochondria also need CoQ10 for proper functioning. This wonderful nutrient has proved its worth in cases of high blood pressure and congestive heart failure (a definite mitochondrial malfunction).

Probiotics: Probiotic supplements help keep a healthy balance of beneficial bacteria in your digestive tract. There are 500 different species of bacteria in the digestive tract; 80 percent are good bacteria and 20 percent are bad bacteria. Good bacteria are critical to your body's ability to deflect incoming toxins so they don't cause overgrowth or imbalance in the digestive tract. The two most plentiful probiotics are lactobacillus, which are primarily found living in the small intestine, and bifidobacterium, most prevalent in your large intestine. When selecting a probiotic supplement, choose a highpotency formula with significant amounts of both bifidobacterium and lactobacillus (culture counts should be in the billions). I recommend taking a good probiotic every day to help maintain a healthy digestive environment in the gut (colon).

When we take antibiotics, many of the body's beneficial bacteria can be killed, which throws off the balance, causing bad bacteria to grow out of control. If you have had repeated rounds of antibiotics to treat illnesses, you could be at risk for developing an overgrowth of intestinal bacteria. Bad bacteria produce endotoxins, which may be as toxic as chemical pesticides or other toxic substances. Although there are yogurt products that are marketed to promote good, healthy bacteria, most of them contain added sugars and are not prepared in a way that allows the most beneficial bacteria to thrive in your digestive tract. So adding yogurt to your diet to get more probiotics is not a bad idea, but I believe that a high-quality probiotic supplement, like PB8, Culturelle, or Ultimate Flora, is most effective.

Vitamin C: Vitamin C is vital for the proper functioning of white blood cells, which fight off the invading bacteria and viruses that lead to colds and flu. Vitamin C also improves the functioning of the enzymes in the liver, helping to eliminate toxins. Vitamin C helps with detoxification and inflammation. Many health practitioners recommend taking 500 to 1,000 mg of buffered ascorbic acid (vitamin C) powder or capsules daily. Personally, I've been taking about 1,000 milligrams of vitamin C for the past ten years with no issues or side effects. I think this is one of the reasons I've gone from getting four to five colds per year to about one per year.

Digestive enzymes: Enzymes break down foods during the digestive process by splitting apart the bonds that hold nutrients together. Enzymes are normally present in raw foods, but many processed and packaged foods are depleted of their natural enzymes through cooking and processing. If the body is lacking essential enzymes needed for proper digestion, the body may not be able to completely break down foods and allow the body to absorb their nutrients. When enzymes in food are destroyed, the digestive organs have to work harder to break down and process that food. So you will want to supplement your diet with digestive enzymes that contain protease, amylase, lipase, and cellulase, which can assist and speed up digestion and the body's absorption of nutrients. After taking them, you will immediately begin to experience less bloating and gas.

Nutritional supplements that improve insulin function and control your blood sugar. In previous section, we discussed how insulin causes weight gain. In this section, I recommend nutritional supplements that have been scientifically proven to lower blood sugar levels, improve insulin function, and reduce appetite and cravings. These nutritional supplements are not weight-loss pills, but if you have insulin resistance, because they work to control your blood sugar and insulin levels, they will cause your body to burn fat and lose weight. If you follow the dietary changes outlined in this book, combined with the recommended nutritional supplements, you will begin to burn fat and become naturally thin.

Alpha-lipoic acid or R-lipoic acid. Alpha-lipoic acid improves insulin function and can gradually decrease blood sugar levels, which helps the body to burn fat. Animal research studies have found that alpha-lipoic acid can reduce appetite, speed up metabolism, and promote weight loss. In addition to being a powerful antioxidant and anti-inflammatory nutrient, alpha-lipoic acid increases the body's ability to take glucose into the cells. This nutrient works synergistically to better regulate blood sugar and insulin levels. Rlipoic acid is a type of lipoic acid that is chemically identical to the one found in nature. R-lipoic acid is more expensive than alpha-lipoic acid, but it can be more effective because it's a more biologically active compound. You can try 100 mg of alpha-lipoic acid or R-lipoic acid about fifteen minutes before each meal, three times a day. However, if you are a diabetic, you can take 200 mg before each meal, three times a day. One of my favorite brands is a product called Insulow. This product combines R-lipoic acid with biotin, both important nutrients for managing insulin resistance and controlling diabetes. Biotin plays a crucial role in managing insulin and blood sugar and is a good supplement to take combined with either chromium or alpha-lipoic-acid or R-lipoic acid.

Chromium: Chromium is a mineral found in the body in trace amounts. Research has shown that chromium supplementation has the ability to even out blood sugar levels while enhancing the body's fat-burning metabolism. Chromium is also known to be helpful in suppressing appetite and cravings. Taking chromium supplements may help control carbohydrate cravings and improve insulin function and glucose metabolism. Research studies have shown that many people with insulin resistance and diabetes have chromium deficiencies; thus, taking chromium supplements can help improve blood glucose levels. Taking chromium supplements in conjunction with eating a healthy diet and engaging in moderate physical activity can result in an outstanding degree of fat burning and weight loss.

There are two leading types of chromium supplements: chromium picolinate and chromium polynicotinate. With the chromium polynicotinate supplement, chromium is bound to a form of the B vitamin, niacin. In the picolinate supplement, chromium is combined with the amino acid tryptophan. There is conflicting information about which type is most effective. Studies have shown that while both types of supplements are safe, chromium polynicotinate is more easily absorbed by the body. There is also more research indicating that chromium polynicotinate promotes fat loss but preserves muscle mass. I have used both types and, for me, chromium picolinate has been much more effective at fat burning and weight loss. However, you should do your research and consult with your doctor to choose which type may be best for you if you suffer from insulin resistance or diabetes. Recommended dosages include 200 to 400 micrograms, three times daily, about fifteen minutes before each meal.

This DHEMM System is the start of a whole new lifestyle. The end goal is to allow you to lose weight, restore your health, and help you transition into a healthy lifestyle of eating and living.

Avoid Foods That Make You Fat

Simply put, certain foods cause you to gain weight more than others do, and these items should be minimized or avoided altogether. The foods listed in this section have the biggest impact on creating excessive fat in the body as well as poor health.

- Sugar

Sugars include refined white sugar, brown sugar, and high-fructose corn syrup. When you eat sugar, you trigger a vicious cycle of sugar cravings, increased insulin production, increased appetite, more sugar intake, and more insulin production, until you are in a cycle of craving, binging, and crashing all day long. Eventually, this leads to insulin resistance, which is a major contributor to weight gain and rapid aging. Examples of foods containing lots of sugar include cakes, pies, candy, barbecue sauce, breakfast cereals, cookies, donuts, fruit punch, fruit juices, ice cream, jellies, pudding, popsicles, sodas, and yogurts with added fruit. Just read the label and look for sugar in the list of ingredients. As a general guideline, try to avoid products that have more than 5 grams of sugar per serving.

- Salt

Many people are aware of the health-related issues, such as high blood pressure and cardiovascular disease, that result from too much salt in their diet. But most people don't realize how salt contributes to weight gain. Salt wreaks havoc on your waistline. A 2007 study published in Obesity Research showed that high-salt diets are directly associated with more fat cells in the body, and even worse, that salt makes fat cells denser and thicker.

When you eat too much salt, your kidneys have to work overtime to excrete the excess. The body can best handle only about 1,400 to 2,500 mg per day, but today most people consume 4,500 to 6,000 mg of salt per day. If the kidneys become unable to excrete all the excess, the salt begins to build up in the tissues and damage cells. When your body has damaged cells, other bodily functions suffer, including the ability to burn fat. A high-salt diet also hardens the arteries, which makes it difficult for oxygen to get to your cells. When you get less oxygen into your cells, you will have a less-efficient metabolism, slowing your ability to burn fat. A high-salt diet makes you retain water and become bloated. Even if you lose body fat, you will remain bloated; you will still look and feel puffy and heavy. Salt attracts and holds water, increasing blood volume and making your body expand and become bigger and thicker. The retention of extra water and fluid results in major bloating. Even after eating a meal high in salt or a salty snack, you'll notice how your stomach begins to look bloated and bigger. Many people with a high-salt diet are carrying around five to ten pounds of extra water weight. When you eat salty snacks, you become thirstier and hungrier and end up overeating—all things you don't want to occur when you're trying to lose weight.

- Trans Fats

There are three types of fats: healthy fats (discussed in the previous section), bad fats (discussed a little later in this section in the section titled "Saturated Fats"), and ugly fats—trans fats, also labeled on products as hydrogenated oils. These manmade fats are the worst of all—considered by many to be toxic. Your body cannot properly digest trans fats, and they negatively impact your weight and health. They are found in fried foods like potato chips, french fries, and onion rings, and, unfortunately, in virtually every commercially packaged or baked good, including cookies, pastries, donuts, and crackers, because they don't spoil quickly and help to extend the shelf life of these products. Eating trans fats is like eating plastic and is very bad for one's health, yet modern Americans consume them in large quantities, often without the slightest awareness of what they are doing. Trans fats disrupt metabolism, cause weight gain, and increase the risk of diabetes, heart disease, inflammation, and cancer.

One Harvard study found that getting just 3 percent of daily calories from trans fats (about 7 to 8 grams of trans fat) increases your risk of heart disease by 50 percent. And given that the average person has about 4 to 10 grams of trans fats in his or her diet, it is no wonder heart disease is such a major killer in modern times. Learn to identify trans fats in foods. Read the labels on all food products before you buy them, and avoid products whose labels contains the words trans-fat, hydrogenated, and partially hydrogenated.

- Saturated Fats

Saturated fats are found in red meat and many dairy products like whole milk, cheese, and butter. Eating a lot of saturated fat can increase cholesterol in your blood and lead to heart attack or stroke. Consumption of these fats should be limited or avoided altogether if possible. To eat less saturated fat, be sure to eat lean meat or skinless poultry, or at least trim the fat before you cook it. You can also eat fewer pastries, cakes, and biscuits—in other words, baked goods that contain butter and/or milk are also high in saturated fats and should be avoided.

- White Flour

White flour, commonly found in many desserts and pastas, contributes to weight gain. Don't let the name "wheat flour" or "enriched wheat flour" fool you. During processing, the two most nutritious parts of the wheat, the bran and the germ, are removed. During the processing from wheat to white flour, many of the nutrients are pulled out of the product. "Wheat flour" or "enriched wheat flour" is essentially the same as white flour, unless the label explicitly lists "whole wheat flour." Whole wheat flour is a healthier alternative. Examples of white flour products that contribute to weight gain include white bread, white pasta, white pizza dough, flour tortillas, biscuits, bread, crackers, crepes, croutons, dumplings, pancakes, piecrust, pretzels, waffles, and noodles. Furthermore, white flour is bleached nearly the same way you bleach your clothing. When you eat white flour, you're eating some of those bleaching agents, which increases the toxic overload in the body.

- Sodas and Sports Drinks

It's possible to consume more calories from sodas and other sweet drinks than from any other single food; there are about 250 calories in one 20- ounce bottle of soda. Sodas are empty calories because they do not provide nutrients. If you are a heavy soda drinker, simply replacing your soda intake with water is a good way to lose a considerable amount of weight within a year. Diet sodas are lower in calories and are a better choice if you are trying to lose weight, even though they have hidden side effects due to the artificial sweeteners used in them. In the previous section, I discussed healthier beverage options.

- Processed Meats

Foods such as hot dogs, salami, pepperoni, bacon, many sausages, etc., are poor-quality meats and are often full of nitrates and other preservatives that are bad for your digestion and health. It's possible to find healthier varieties of these foods that do not contain nitrates or preservatives in stores like Whole Foods or at butcher shops. If you do need to splurge once in a while by having bacon or sausage, find these less-processed, healthier varieties.

- Cow's Milk Products

Milk that you think does the body good may actually be contributing to the deterioration of your bones and organs. Cow's milk is too difficult for the human body to break down, which means it will leave waste residue in the body that piles up over time if consumed on a regular basis. Just as breast milk is designed for human infants, cow's milk is designed for baby cows, not for us. Additionally, because the milk is pasteurized, most of its positive attributes, like its enzymes, are cooked out. It is true that dairy products contain calcium, but they also contain animal proteins that are very difficult for the body to digest. And calcium can be obtained from other food sources, such as nuts, seeds, and green leafy veggies like kale, spinach, and dandelion greens, which are high in absorbable calcium and also provide many other essential nutrients.

Another problem with cow's milk is that the cows are injected with growth hormones and antibiotics to help them produce milk, and we take those hormones and antibiotics directly into our bloodstream when we consume milk products. Because milk is considered a high mucus-forming food, it leads to allergies, infections, colds, and asthma—ailments many kids experience because they consume more milk products than adults do.

Children end up with mucus buildup very early in their life. Dairy products made from the milk of goats and sheep are better than those made from cow's milk, particularly if they are raw. There are also nondairy milk options, such as almond, rice, hemp, or soy milk (unsweetened). The natural enzymes in goat's milk are far closer to those in humans, so we're able to digest goat's milk significantly better. If you love cheese, consider switching to goat cheese, particularly in its raw, unpasteurized form, which can be a good treat for you. Sheep's milk cheese is the next best choice. If you still decide to consume products made with cow's milk, buy organic and fat-free or low-fat brands because they are more nutritious.

Diet Foods That Make You Fat

There are many products marketed as "diet" because they have some reduced amount of sugar or fat. But without looking at all the ingredients, you won't be able to identify the hidden ones that may contribute to weight gain. Also, there are many low-calorie products that have little to no nutritional value and provide very little health benefit.

- Diet Sodas

Although diet sodas are better than regular sodas because they have no sugar, diet sodas still cause some health and weight issues. The artificial sweeteners in diet sodas are thought to potentially cause some health problems, including cancer. Have you ever wondered why people walk around all day drinking diet sodas but they are not thin? Diet sodas are made from chemicals and have no nutritional value. When the body finds nothing recognizable as nutrition, the brain sends signals to be fed something nutritional, which creates cravings for more. Diet sodas make you crave fattening foods. If you are addicted to sodas and diet sodas, you could drink green tea, which is a fat burner and helps you lose more weight while still getting your caffeine fix for the day. You could also try plain water. If plain water does not sound appealing, try adding a bit of lemon or cranberry juice to it. However, don't replace soda with a lot of store-bought juices, because they contain a lot of sugar and additives that cause weight gain.

- Sugar-Free Baked Goods

You have to be careful that sugar-free baked goods don't have the same amount of or more fat than the original recipes. Although the serving size may say 0 grams of sugar, it could very well have 9 grams of fat, which can also cause weight gain. Until you totally wean yourself off sugar and sweets, to satisfy your sweet tooth, try graham crackers, which have less sugar (about a teaspoon less per serving than most other cookies) and very little fat, about 2 grams per serving. They provide a subtle sweetness without the tremendous number of calories contained in cakes and cookies.

- Fat-Free Dressings

Trying to avoid fats altogether should not be the goal. There are healthy fats that are very good for the body. Most fat-free products are generally higher in sugar, which defeats the overall purpose of eating a fat-free product to lose weight. Try an oil-based, reduced-fat dressing that contains olive or canola oil (healthy fats) and has 2 to 4 grams of fat per serving.

- High-Protein Diet Bars (Power Bars) and Shakes

When the body receives a protein or power bar, it tries to break down the sugar and chemicals in it, but when these elements cannot be fully digested by the body, the excess ends up being stored in the body as fat. A better alternative is an avocado, which is high in protein, and because it is in its natural state, the body knows how to break it down completely and use it to fuel the body.

- Fruit Snacks

Fruit snacks have added sugars and artificial ingredients that counteract any potential nutritional benefits they might have. Don't get fooled by marketing if the package says the product is made with real fruit or fruit juices. Instead, read the list of ingredients on the nutrition label; if the product has a high number of grams of sugar, it is fattening. A better alternative is to eat fresh fruit. Just get the real thing and gain all the benefits of fruits. Unlike fruit snacks, real fruit is rich in fiber, phytonutrients, and cancer-fighting antioxidants. You should even watch out for dried fruit because it usually contains a lot of added sugar as well.

- Artificial Sweeteners

You know them in those little yellow, pink, and blue packages that are generally marketed as "sugar substitutes." Most people don't realize that even though artificial sweeteners generally have zero calories, they can still contribute to weight gain. These artificial sweeteners increase appetite by sending false signals to the brain that sweet food is on the way. The brain subsequently becomes confused when sweet food never arrives and so it never gives the signal that you are satisfied. You develop a sweet tooth and sugar cravings throughout the day, sometimes causing you to eat more sugar. Let's look at aspartame, in particular. Despite its zero calories, studies have shown that aspartame can, in fact, induce weight gain. Some researchers believe that the two main ingredients in aspartame, phenylalanine and aspartic acid, stimulate the release of insulin and leptin, hormones that instruct our bodies to store fat, according to a study called "Physiological Mechanisms Mediating Aspartame-Induced Satiety."

The best choice for a calorie-free sweetener is stevia, an herb that grows naturally in parts of Paraguay and Brazil and is now widely available in this country. You don't need much of it—according to studies, it's thirty times sweeter than sugar. Yet it does not raise blood sugar levels or cause rapidonset cravings the way simple sugars do. A study published in the Journal of Ethno-Pharmacology found that stevia dilates the blood vessels and helps to prevent high blood pressure. It also helps to regulate the digestive system, encourages the growth of friendly bacteria, and helps us detoxify the body and excrete more urine naturally. Just because a product is labeled low-fat or fat free doesn't always mean the product is not still high in sugar, salt, and calories. You should get in the habit of reading food labels to ensure the product is healthy and nutritional. However, if you limit or avoid the food items listed above, you will have a much easier time getting to your ideal weight.

Scott J. Barnard

CHAPTER 3

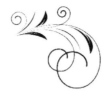

THE DHEMM SYSTEM: A PERMANENT WEIGHT-LOSS SYSTEM

The DHEMM System addresses the underlying causes of weight gain, which are:

- Toxic overload
- Hormonal imbalances
- Sluggish metabolism
- Unhealthy eating habits

The DHEMM System provides a quick-start plan for dramatically but naturally addressing all of the above factors in your efforts to lose weight and improve your health. You should look forward to an exciting journey. The DHEMM System is not a temporary solution to weight loss. Expect your life to change for the better because you will not only lose weight, have more energy, and look better; you will likely, for the first time ever, desire healthy, nutrient-rich foods.

The DHEMM System will provide your body with foods, supplements, and detox methods that help the body get rid of toxins, correct hormonal imbalances, and crave healthy foods. Your body does the rest automatically. It has a natural ability to heal and restore balance; the body can renew and rejuvenate itself naturally. Your body's natural intelligence does know what to do if you simply get out of the way. If you give it a rest and a chance to repair and heal, it will. Also, by eliminating the major sources of foods that introduce toxins and cause disease, such as sugar and flour products, bad fats/oils, and food allergens, your body can heal itself.

The DHEMM System focuses on good nutrition and healthy eating. You will learn what to eat and how to make your body burn fat more efficiently while controlling cravings and hunger. You will learn which foods actually boost your metabolism and target excess fat in the body. The focus of the DHEMM System revolves around "super foods" that detoxify and cleanse the body of fat while also providing the highest sources of protein, carbs, and fiber that help the pounds melt away.

Following the DHEMM System will provide you with these benefits:

• You will flush away waste and excess fat quickly and learn how to keep your body fat-resistant for years to come.

• You will remove years from your face as fine lines and wrinkles diminish, allowing you to experience a "second youth."

• You will experience weight loss due to the elimination of excess waste. Impacted fecal matter in your colon and digestive system cause excess weight in the body.

• You will have more energy as your body responds better to healthy foods. By removing excess waste, your body will absorb even more nutrients from the foods you eat, leaving you feeling energized and well.

• You will see a decrease in feelings of indigestion, bloating, and fatigue after eating.

• You will learn new ways to make time for sleep, rest, and relaxation and simple, easy ways to get moving and speed up your metabolism without going to a gym.

• You will get rid of unhealthy cravings. By changing your eating habits for just one month, you will become aware of how different foods affect you, allowing you to begin avoiding foods that are bad for you.

• You will feel more balanced and happy due to a healthy balance among your body's hormonal signals.

What you won't get on the DHEMM System are the following:

• Calorie counting: There will be no calorie counting or measuring grams of food.

• Exercise regimen: You won't have to exercise in the gym for hours a week (unless you choose to do so for the other health benefits exercise provides).

• Going hungry: You shouldn't experience severe hunger during this program if you follow my recommendations.

• Cravings: Although you may experience cravings during the first phase, you shouldn't expect them after that. It is necessary to break the addiction to many unhealthy foods that you've been eating for so long.

• Bland, boring foods: You also don't have to worry about disgusting or tasteless food. The food choices are delicious, with plenty of options to choose from.

• Slow results: People often complain that it takes too long to see the benefits and get results from traditional diets, but you can expect rapid weight loss on the DHEMM System.

Whenever I'm planning a long vacation or trip, I take time to find a nice hotel, get a flight, and pick out the clothes I want to wear. In other words, I take time to get ready. The same is true for the journey toward health and wellness on which you are about to embark. Take time to properly prepare for the program. It will make your transition easier, and you will be more likely to succeed in following the program. Spend several days preparing to begin the DHEMM System. Gather the foods, supplies, supplements, and any additional resources (e.g., books). You may even want to cut back on foods that will be eliminated during the detox phase, such as caffeine, sugar, sodas, processed or packaged junk and fast foods, and white-flour products, a few days before you begin. Eliminating items from your diet in a systematic way will help minimize potential withdrawal symptoms and jump-start the process to weight loss and optimal health.

An Overview of the Five Key Elements of the DHEMM System

DHEMM stands for Detox, Hormonal Balance, Eat, Mental Mastery, and Move. The system focuses on helping you detoxify, cleanse, and reset your taste buds so that you desire healthy, natural foods. Each of the five key elements of the program includes detoxification methods, food and beverage choices, and supplements to enhance your progress.

D is for DETOX: Get rid of toxins in the body for fast weight loss. You will detoxify the body through elimination of certain foods for three weeks, as well as use other detoxification methods that eliminate toxic waste from your body. As you do this, you will get rid of unhealthy foods and reprogram your taste buds to desire healthy, nutrient-rich foods.

H is for HORMONAL BALANCE: As I discussed earlier, hormones control your appetite, metabolism, and how much weight you gain or lose. With the DHEMM system, we address the hormones that impact our weight and health, and provide tips for balancing our hormones for optimum health and weight loss.

E is for EAT: Eat "clean and balanced" foods for permanent weight loss. You will learn the method of eating clean and balanced foods to help you achieve your ideal weight. You will enjoy the healthy, whole-food eating plan you started in the detoxification phase but will begin to reintroduce some of the foods you avoided and determine which ones will have negative consequences on your health or weight-loss efforts. When reintroducing them, you can monitor their effects on your health. As an example, if you drink milk and find that you get a stuffy nose, it is best that you stay away from milk because it is creating intolerances in your system.

M is for MOVE: Get moving without going to the gym or "working out." You can begin this part of the program right away. I will help you incorporate easy and effective ways of getting physically active, as well as strengthening your muscles, into your everyday life.

M is for MENTAL MASTERY: I begin to discuss motivation and mental mastery—weight loss starts in the mind before it starts in the body. It's important that we have the right mental focus to achieve our long-term weight-loss goals.

I've designed this five-phase system with not only your body in mind but also your overall health and well-being. You will get rid of excess fat in your body and reverse some of your health issues and ailments, restoring your body to optimal health. Now that it has become easier and more economical to get access to better-quality organic foods and supplements, optimal health is achievable for everyone. We can find most of what we need right in our grocery store.

There are many large and small changes that you can make in your lifestyle and diet that have an immediate impact and enormous improvement on your health. However you go about doing the DHEMM System, the journey will be uniquely yours, and the changes you experience will be perfect and appropriate for you.

Detox (D) — Get Rid Of Toxins For Fast Weight Loss

The DHEMM System is geared for weight loss as well as detoxification. You will get the benefits of weight loss, but more importantly, you will transition to living a healthier, more vibrant life. This detox phase is designed to transition you to eating whole, unprocessed, natural foods as well as removing the most common unhealthy food choices. During this phase, you are reeducating your body and programming your taste buds to enjoy foods that help you lose weight and keep it off. You will also eliminate foods to which you may have sensitivities that cause inflammation in the body. It is not uncommon to lose up to fifteen pounds in this three-week phase. Besides weight loss, you can expect to feel more energetic, to sleep better, and to be rid of chronic sinus and digestive problems and recurring headaches.

In this phase, you will begin the cleansing process by focusing on foods that cleanse and detoxify the body, while avoiding foods that cause weight gain, excess toxins, and inflammation in the body. You will reprogram your taste buds to crave whole, natural, healthy foods as opposed to high-sugar junk foods. You will begin to enjoy a new variety of foods while still losing weight during this three-week period. During this phase, you will be eliminating the Big 6, the most addictive, unhealthy, and fattening foods. At the end of the three weeks, when you can begin to reintroduce these foods, you will likely have lost your taste for them. Once your body doesn't crave them, you will have a balanced body chemistry that lets you eat them in moderation, from time to time, but not every day.

You will be reprogramming your body to enjoy and crave natural and healthy foods that limit insulin production in the body, which is an underlying cause of excess fat in the body. You will also eat foods that build and maintain muscle tone with very little effort. In choosing what to eat, you will balance carbohydrates, proteins, and fats at every meal. You will not be counting calories: the focus is on quality of calories, not quantity. Consuming large amounts of fresh vegetables, fruits, grains, beans, nuts, seeds, and fats will rebuild your cells following detox. If you love to eat like I do, you will be glad to know that for the three weeks of this phase, you will enjoy eating delicious, nutrient-rich foods and you won't be hungry. Don't worry about failing or giving up if discipline is not your strong suit. Here's what you do. If you slip up or eat some of the foods you're supposed to avoid, just continue to avoid the Big 6 foods and keep pressing forward. Challenge yourself to stick to the program, but don't beat yourself up too badly if you slip up. If you find that one or two items, like coffee, is too difficult to give up, just avoid everything but caffeine and make the most of the program anyway. That is still better than giving up entirely. Maybe the next time you try it, you'll be ready to give up all of the Big 6 foods. It's all about making good progress, not being perfect! Another option is to find a friend, coworker, or family member to follow the DHEMM System with you so you can support and encourage one another. This is your journey. Make it your own, enjoy it, and make it appropriate for you.

Big 6 Foods to Avoid During This Phase

In this phase, you will avoid the following Big 6 foods and beverages for three weeks. The Big 6 foods to avoid are either fattening, addictive, and/or unhealthy. The Big 6 foods to avoid are:

1. Caffeine drinks (tea, coffee, soda, diet soda)
2. Sugar (candy, sweets, cookies, cakes, processed foods that contain sugar)
3. White Carbs (white bread, white rice, white pasta, white potatoes)
4. Animal Proteins (eggs, fish, chicken, beef)
5. Dairy (milk and cheese)
6. Alcohol (liquor, beer, wine)

In this phase, I recommend that you abstain from the Big 6 for three weeks and replace them with healthy, whole, plant-based foods, such as nutritious vegetables, whole grains, beans, fruits, and nuts. When people decide to refrain from eating the Big 6, the first thing they ask me is, "What in the world is left to eat?" But you'll discover a whole array of delicious, natural foods that make you feel healthy and energetic. You won't have to starve or feel hungry because you will be eating—just different foods than your body is used to eating. As in the entire DHEMM System, you will not be counting calories or measuring carbs, proteins, or fats, just learning to enjoy healthier foods that will fuel your body. Also, if you are satisfied with the food choices and your weight loss during this phase, you can continue in it as long as you like as it has very healthy, natural food choices. However, for those who want to begin to add some of the Big 6 foods back into their diet, progressing to the next phase will guide you toward a long-term, healthy eating plan.

Foods to Eat During This Phase

To ensure you get the highest-quality foods, you may have to visit a local health food store, not just a regular grocery store. A local health food store will have more natural, organic foods with more options as well. I personally never thought I would crave raw seeds and nuts, but I just love them for an afternoon snack, particularly sunflower seeds and cashews. They sure beat the candy I'd eat after raiding the vending machine most afternoons before I began the DHEMM System.

Breakfast Foods
• Whole grain or mixed grain cereals: There are a variety of hot and cold cereals that contain whole grain or mixed grain. Oatmeal is a great choice, and you can use stevia or fresh fruit to sweeten to taste.

Lunch/Dinner Foods
• Vegetables: A few good choices include spinach, kale, collard greens, broccoli, cauliflower, green beans, asparagus, Brussels sprouts, zucchini, eggplant, squash, tomatoes, and mushrooms.
• Whole grains: Brown or wild rice, whole grain crackers, buckwheat, quinoa.
• Salads: Make yourself luxurious salads using mixed greens, romaine lettuce, spinach, arugula, carrots, mushrooms, cucumber, radicchio, endive, peppers, avocado, tomato, and radishes.
• Beans and legumes: Though they are considered starches, beans and legumes are especially healthy kinds because they are high in fiber and low in fat. Go wild eating black beans, lima beans, kidney beans, fava beans, butter beans, lentils, chickpeas, and black-eyed peas. Canned beans are fine, but you may want to rinse some of the salt off them before cooking.

• Tofu, tempeh, and faux meats: Sauté, bake, or grill tofu and tempeh, and mix them with vegetables and brown rice. There are also good vegetarian meat substitutes for burgers, sausage, or chicken patties available.

Snacks

• Fruits: A few good choices include apples, blackberries, blueberries, raspberries, strawberries, cherries, peaches, goji berries, grapefruits, and oranges.

• Nuts and seeds: These include almonds, walnuts, macadamia nuts, cashews, soy nuts, sunflower seeds, pumpkin seeds, sesame seeds, hemp seeds, and freshly ground flaxseeds, just to name a few. Buy organic raw nuts and seeds when possible.

• Other snack choices: Rice cakes, flax crackers, unsweetened peanut butter, and popcorn (lightly seasoned with sea salt is fine).

Cooking Ingredients

• Cooking oils: The best choices are extra-virgin olive oil, organic canola, sunflower, and safflower oils, and walnut oil.

• Seasonings: Use Celtic Sea salt, garlic, onions, ginger, and tamari. Do not use regular table salt.

• Oils to use on salads: The best choices are flaxseed oil, avocado oil, and olive oil.

• Gluten-free flours: Good choices are flours that contain rice, beans, oats, soy, barley, potato, cornmeal, flaxseed, nuts, seeds, quinoa, or tapioca.

• Non-dairy butters: Use nut or seed butters, such as almond butter, or vegan butter. Be sure the butters are unsweetened.

• Sweeteners: Stevia is especially good for cereals, smoothies, and baked goods. Agave nectar is another option to use in moderation.

Beverages

In the previous section, I discussed some of the best beverage options and explained the specific health benefits they provide. The recommended beverages to drink during this phase are listed below:

- Water
- Coconut water
- Fresh-squeezed juices
- Herbal caffeine-free teas like mint or chamomile
- Non-dairy milk, such as unsweetened almond, rice, hemp, or soy milk

Detoxification Methods That Support This Phase

Detoxifying the body and eliminating toxins can be accomplished through various detoxification methods. During this three week detoxification phase, I consider it mandatory that you take colon cleansing and liver cleansing herbs/supplements. You need to rapidly eliminate toxins from your body to avoid feeling sick and to minimize detox symptoms. All the other detox methods listed are optional, but I would strongly encourage you to pick two or three of the others on a long-term basis, as you have the time and money to do so. Some people notice a change for the better in their health and energy levels within a few days; however, for others, it may take a few months.

Everyone's toxic overload is different, and many factors come into play, such as your health status, weight, metabolism, age, and genetics. So be patient and steadfast through the detoxification process.

What to Expect During This Phase

You may be surprised at how good you feel after this phase—lighter and more energetic. You may experience greater mental clarity. Many people who thought being sluggish and lethargic was a normal way of living are pleasantly surprised at how great they feel. As a result of this detox phase, you will have given your body a chance to break free from cravings and addictive eating habits. You may have some cravings, and there may be some days when the process will seem difficult, but you will begin to see the light at the end of the tunnel. Some individuals don't experience any cravings at all.

Expect and Welcome Detox Symptoms

You may experience some detoxification symptoms, and their severity will depend on how toxic you were to begin with. You should expect and welcome detox symptoms because, although they can be unpleasant, they are a sign of progress. Your body is addicted to the Big 6 foods, and as you break those addictions, you will be learning for the first time how dependent your body has become on those foods.

Typical detox symptoms include the following:

• Cravings: As your body detoxifies, it craves foods it was used to eating, such as meat, dairy, sugar, and caffeine. Cravings may last for several hours or several days, but they will begin to decrease as your body gets rid of its toxic overload.

• Headaches, pains, nausea: If you drink a lot of coffee, expect headaches during the first few days. You may also experience physical aches and joint pains or even nausea.

• Fatigue: Allow time to rest during this detoxification phase, as eliminating toxins will drain you and make you feel exhausted. Just take it easy and rest.

• Skin rashes: Skin rashes, or even acne, are signs that your body is excreting toxins through your skin, which is the body's largest organ of elimination. By doing the colonics or taking the colon-cleansing herbs, you can minimize the rashes and breakouts.

• Irritability: Not eating some of your favorite foods will make you feel irritable and bored, so expect to be a little cranky. This is a good time to avoid social events as well.

The body is fully capable of healing, rejuvenating, and restoring itself to optimum health, and detoxification allows you to do just that. The twenty-one days should give your body sufficient time to reprogram your taste buds, and you will begin to enjoy healthier, more natural foods, permanently changing your unhealthy eating habits. After the twenty-one days of this detoxification phase, you will experience great health benefits. You will begin to naturally slim down. You will begin to think more clearly. You will feel energized and more alive. You will notice a clearer complexion. You will feel happier and balanced. And, most important, detoxifying the body on a long-term basis will ensure your body doesn't accumulate toxic waste that leads to excess fat in the body.

Eat (E) — Eat Clean And Balanced Foods For Permanent Weight Loss

In earlier section, we discussed which foods are healthy and contribute to weight gain and which ones contribute to weight loss. In this section, we focus on how much to eat, what types of food, and what combinations of foods are best for the body. You will enjoy the healthy, whole-food eating plan you started in the detoxification phase but will begin to reintroduce some of the foods you avoided and determine which ones will have negative consequences on your health or weight-loss efforts. When reintroducing them, you can monitor their effects on your health. As you begin to reintroduce certain foods, you will need to observe how they affect your weight and how you feel. If certain foods still cause you to have allergic reactions (bloating, gas, headaches) and hinder your weight-loss goals, you will want to continue to avoid them. You may want to keep a journal at this time to keep track of what you eat every day and the feelings or allergic symptoms associated with certain foods.

The foods in the DHEMM System will help you balance hormones, decrease hunger, regulate your metabolism, and remove toxins that lead to chronic disease. The foods in the DHEMM System, which include lean proteins, good carbs, and healthy fats at each meal, have the following characteristics:

- Low in sugar
- Primarily natural, whole, raw, or organic
- High in fiber and omega-3 fatty acids
- High in vitamins, minerals, and nutrients
- Low in sodium

Transitioning from the Detox Phase to the Eat Phase

Here are a few key guidelines to help you transition from the Detox Phase to the Eat Phase. This will help ensure that you continue to lose weight as you transition to the Eat Phase. Regarding the Big 6 Foods that you avoided in Phase 1 (Detox Phase), here's how you should transition these foods back into your diet:

1. Caffeine drinks: Feel free to add a limited amount of caffeine back into your diet. Caffeine can speed up your metabolism by 5 to 8 percent, which helps to burn about 100 to 175 calories a day. This does not mean you should overdo it and drink several cups of coffee per day, but having one cup of coffee will not have adverse effects on your weight-loss goals. Additionally, green tea, my favorite metabolism booster, is found to provide many health benefits to the body as well as help your body burn fat. Green tea is highly recommended as a daily drink.

2. Sugar: I explained that sugar is highly addictive and how it makes us fat and sick; there is no good reason to bring sugar back into your diet. Of course, we are referring to white refined sugar, high fructose corn syrup, etc. You should

continue to use stevia and other natural sweeteners that don't have adverse effects on your health and weight-loss goals.

3. White carbs: You will continue to avoid white carbs, such as white bread, white rice, white pasta, white flour, and white potatoes. Feel free to use healthier alternatives, such as whole grain bread, brown or wild rice, whole grain pasta, whole wheat flours, and sweet potatoes.

4. Meats: Meats provide the body with lean proteins, which are extremely effective for helping to maintain muscle, burn calories, and balance blood sugar levels. So, during this phase, you want to transition meats (lean protein) back into your diet. A good approach is to bring back fish for the first week, then bring back chicken, and the following week, you can have lean red meat on occasion. Red meat contains a lot of saturated fat, so try to limit your intake to two or three times a week. Instead, eat more protein from fish, poultry, and vegetable sources, such as brown rice, beans, and nuts.

5. Dairy: If you discovered that you're allergic to dairy (cow's milk) during the Detox Phase, then you want to continue avoiding it. However, eggs, low-fat cheese, and non-dairy milk (such as almond milk or soy milk) are still great long-term dairy options.

6. Alcohol: If you were a drinker before the Detox Phase, you're probably anxious to bring alcohol back into your diet. However, you should still drink alcohol in moderation. Be mindful how harsh alcohol can be on the liver; you will want to do liver cleanses every few months if you consume a great deal of alcohol.

Detox Methods: In the Detox Phase, you completed a colon cleanse and a liver cleanse. For maintenance, you can do colon cleansing and liver cleansing as you feel a toxic overload building up in your system, and, for most, this is typically every three to six months. However, for those who maintain healthy eating, drink clean or alkaline water, or take few to no prescriptions or supplements, you may only need to do colon or liver cleansing once a year.

Supplements: In the Detox Phase, the green drink and fiber were mandatory supplements. You can continue both of these supplements, as they will continue to help you improve your health, cleanse your digestive tract, and help you achieve your weight-loss goals. During this phase, you also want to consider adding any additional supplements. Keep in mind that these supplements are not required but can be added to address specific ailments and digestive issues.

One Final Note: You must understand the difference between "body fat" and "stubborn body fat." You can burn body fat by eating healthy "clean and balanced" meals and being physically active, but to lose stubborn body fat, you will have to correct hormonal imbalances, as discussed in Section 6. When eating healthy and being physically active are not enough to achieve your weight-loss goals, hormonal imbalances are the likely culprit. If you are challenged to lose weight or your weight loss stalls, you will have to incorporate methods to balance your hormones. Additionally, be sure you've include some of the metabolism boosters to help your body burn more fat effortlessly.

What Are "Clean and Balanced" Foods?

As discussed earlier, "clean" foods are primarily natural, whole, raw, or organic—foods that the body can effectively digest and utilize for energy without leaving excess waste or toxins in the body. Clean foods include lean proteins, good carbs, and healthy fats. "Balanced" foods means that you will balance your meals by eating protein every time you eat a carbohydrate. So, if you have carbohydrates, you want to always include protein. Maintaining this balance between proteins and carbs is a very simple but incredibly effective method for preventing insulin spikes and aiding the body in burning fat.

Why protein every time you eat? Protein counteracts the body's overreaction to carbohydrates, which cause insulin spikes and fat storage. Proteins will also help you feel full longer and thus will help prevent overeating and food cravings. Protein will also help you build and maintain muscle mass, and, as we've learned, muscle naturally burns more calories than fat.

Eating clean and balanced foods will help you lose weight for all of the following reasons.

- It will help you address the underlying reasons your body stores fat.
- You will learn which foods will help you stay thin and maintain your healthy weight.
- You will have more control over your insulin and blood sugar levels.
- You will burn fat, especially the belly fat and love handles.
- You will gain control of your appetite and cravings.

Twelve Principles for Eating "Clean and Balanced" Foods

Look at the principles below as your instructions on how to eat "clean and balanced" foods.

• Principle #1: Choose nutrient-rich foods, not empty calories. This means you will eat foods that are high in vitamins, minerals, phytonutrients, fiber, and omega-3 fatty acids. Eating junk foods is like eating empty calories. You want your calories to provide you with nutritional benefits that will help you heal your body and maintain a permanently healthy weight. Before you eat anything, ask yourself, Is this a healthy, nutrient-rich food or empty calories? Commit to be mindful of everything you eat.

• Principle #2: Eat protein with every meal. Eat protein with every meal, and eat it first, before the carbohydrates or fats. You can also eat protein by itself. Eating protein foods does not cause insulin spikes, making them an important staple of eating clean and balanced foods.

• Principle #3: Always balance carbohydrates with protein. Whenever you eat a carbohydrate, eat some protein along with it. As a general guideline, the protein should be about half the amount of the carbohydrates. For example, if you had 30 grams of carbohydrates, then eat about 15 grams of protein along with it to prevent insulin spikes that cause excess fat to be stored in the body. You can use food labels to determine how much carbs (or "net carbs") and protein is in food. (See the examples at the end of this section to better understand how to balance carbohydrates with protein at each meal.)

• Principle #4: Don't overeat carbohydrates. It is important to not overeat carbohydrates. Limit yourself to no more than two servings of high-carbohydrate foods at any one meal or snack. This will prevent excess carbohydrates from being stored as fat. If you are still hungry, then eat more vegetables to satisfy your hunger. Do not try to eat other high-carbohydrate foods, which will convert to fat in your body, or too much protein, which will hinder weight loss by adding extra calories. One serving of high-carbohydrate foods is about 1/2 cup or 15 grams of carbohydrates. So, the maximum amount of high-carb foods you should eat at any one meal is two servings, which is 30 grams or about 1 cup, always balanced with a high-protein food.

• Principle #5: Avoid sugar, salt, and trans fat. We discussed a number of foods that cause weight gain and are bad for your health. However, these three are at the top of the list. Try to avoid them at all costs. They have no nutritional value and are simply bad for your health. Previous section is entirely devoted to explaining how detrimental sugar is. Salt is also bad for your health and causes bloating, swelling, and fluid retention. As far as trans-fat, the good news is that the FDA regulates it, and food manufacturers now have to list how much trans-fat is in each serving when trans fats exceed 0.5 gram per serving.

• Principle #6: Eat at least five servings of fruits and veggies each day. Fruit breaks down faster in the body than any other food, leaving us fueled and energized, and because it is a highly cleansing food, it leaves no toxic residue and acts as a strong cleanser for the body. You need to eat vegetables if you want to get thin, as studies have shown that those who eat a large variety of vegetables have the least amount of body fat. Veggies and fruits are naturally balanced because they contain both protein and carbohydrates. They are made up of mostly water and fiber, so they can be eaten in larger quantities. However, there are a few exceptions. Consumption of corn and potatoes should be minimal and, of course, always be balanced with protein.

• Principle #7: Limit your intake of red meat to two to three times per week. Red meat contains a lot of saturated fat, so try to limit your intake to two or three times a week. Instead, eat more protein from fish, poultry, and vegetable sources, such as brown rice, beans, and nuts, which contain good essential fats.

• Principle #8: Eat two healthy snacks per day. Snacks keep you from getting hungry between meals. Eating snacks allows you to feed your body every three to four hours, which keeps your metabolism revved up. See the list of healthy snacks provided later in this section.

• Principle #9: Eat at least 30 grams of fiber per day. Numerous studies have shown that high-fiber diets help you lose weight and protect against heart disease, stroke, and certain kinds of cancer. It provides a list of foods that are high in fiber as well as fiber supplements that help you to eat 30 grams of fiber per day.

• Principle #10: Eat fruit by itself, one hour before or after meals. The enzymes in fruit are digested better if the fruit is eaten alone. Therefore, fruit is a perfect snack food.

• Principle #11: Eat four to five times a day. You will lose weight more quickly if you eat four or five times a day as opposed to only three meals (or fewer). Try to eat every three to four hours, and think in terms of three meals and two healthy snacks. Each time you eat, you stimulate your metabolism for a short period of time; thus, the more often you eat, the more you speed up your metabolism. Eating every two to three hours feeds your muscles and starves fat.

• Principle #12: Buy organic as much as possible. Buy organic foods, which don't have chemical preservatives, food additives, hormones, pesticides, or antibiotics. Fresh organic foods are far less toxic than highly processed and packaged/frozen foods and leave less residue and waste in the body.

Beverages to Drink During This Phase

The beverages allowed during this phase include water, green tea, freshsqueezed juices, green smoothies, coconut water, non-dairy milk options, an occasional diet soda if desired, and possibly a cup of coffee a day. During periods of intense detoxification (like in Phase 1), I have abstained from drinking coffee, but at other times, I do enjoy drinking a cup a day. There are different schools of thought on whether coffee is bad for our health. Although coffee is acid forming, it is not too harsh on the liver; therefore, in my opinion, it will not interfere with your detoxification and cleansing steps for the long term. However, in the first phase of the DHEMM System, coffee should be avoided altogether. Eventually, you may find you desire less. In any case, coffee is not the biggest problem with staying slim and healthy. If you have a moderate amount of caffeine (about two cups of coffee or tea per day) and can sleep well at night and maintain energy and balance throughout the day, then caffeine may actually improve your health and metabolic fitness. I also recommend drinking green tea instead of coffee because it offers so many other health benefits. But if one (just one) cup of coffee (regular or decaf) in the morning is your guilty pleasure, then that should not pose a problem to your health.

Detox Methods and Supplements That Support This Phase

All of the mandatory detox methods and supplements should be continued during this phase. You will want to continue trying different detox methods to identify those that are most effective for you. Additionally, you will want to consider taking nutritional supplements based upon your specific health concerns and issues. As an example, if you struggle with constipation or bloating, in addition to the green drink and fiber, probiotics and digestive enzymes would be good options to include during this phase.

• Reintroducing Foods and Identifying Food Allergies

During this phase, you can begin introducing the foods that you were avoiding in Phase 1, but be aware of what is going on in your body during this time. During Phase 1 of the program, you may have eliminated foods you were unknowingly sensitive or even allergic to, and thus reintroducing these foods will trigger the symptoms those foods caused you to have. Food allergies are not just the dramatic reactions that cause someone to end up in an emergency room with hives and shortness of breath from peanuts or something like that. That is an immediate and acute allergic reaction. It is not that common but can be very serious. However, there are reactions to foods that are much less dramatic but just as deadly. These are delayed allergies, and they are much more common, affecting millions of people. They are not easily diagnosed but they play a huge role in chronic illness and weight issues. About half of us have some foods that just don't agree with us and that cause a delayed allergic reaction. These delayed allergic reactions can cause symptoms anywhere from a few hours to several days after consumption. These delayed allergic reactions include weight gain, fluid retention, skin eruptions, fatigue, brain fog, irritable bowel syndrome, mood problems, headaches, sinus and nasal congestion, and muscle and joint pain or swelling. Eating foods you are allergic to causes inflammation, which ultimately leads to swelling and fluid retention. Getting rid of this fluid by reducing inflammation is a good thing and can happen with the detoxification methods described in this book. Your body can then start the healing process to allow you to achieve permanent weight loss and optimal health.

The foods most people are sensitive to are gluten, cow's milk, eggs, corn, peanuts, yeast, and wheat. Gluten is a special type of protein that is commonly found in rye, wheat, and barley and is responsible for the elastic texture of dough. It is found in most types of cereals and in many types of bread. Not all foods from the grain family contain gluten. Examples of grains that do not have gluten include wild rice, corn, buckwheat, millet, quinoa, oats, and soybeans. Because gluten is not a naturally occurring protein in the human body, studies have shown that it can cause general inflammation of the intestinal tract and can also damage the lining of the small intestine, making it difficult to absorb nutrients from foods. Eliminating food allergies is the foundation for feeling better and dealing with chronic symptoms. To determine what foods you're allergic to, you can take a blood test for immunoglobulin G (IgG) antibodies to foods. This can be helpful but may not detect all food allergies. It may be more useful for you to identify food allergies by the process of elimination. This simply means you get rid of all potential foods that you think you may be allergic to for three or four weeks and then reintroduce them slowly, one at a time, and see how your system reacts to each one. Keep a food journal and take notes on how different foods affect how you feel or what symptoms they cause in your body. Write down what you eat, when you ate it, and how you felt for the next couple of days after you ate it. A journal will also record your overall weight loss and health and well-being. For example, if you are trying to determine if you are allergic to wheat, you could eat a serving of Wheatena at breakfast and maybe a sandwich with wheat bread for lunch. Then observe your body carefully for the next two to three days. Watch to see if the wheat triggers any symptoms such as fluid retention, headaches, runny nose, or joint pain. If you experience such reactions or symptoms after you reintroduce the food, do not continue to include that food in your diet. Instead, wait and retry again in another month or two. If you still react negatively, you should just remove them from your diet altogether or visit a dietitian or nutritionist skilled in managing food allergies. Because the foods we're most allergic or sensitive to are the ones we eat daily and crave, avoiding these foods can initially be a challenge. You should expect withdrawal symptoms and cravings for the addictive foods for only three to four days. Additionally, any of the allergic reactions could worsen during that time frame. However, after those few days, you will feel better and begin to experience a sense of well-being. Symptoms such as brain fog, fluid retention, low energy, bloating, headaches, and other digestive complaints will lessen as well. Once you eliminate the offending foods, you allow your body to respond more efficiently to the rest of this program, and healing and weight loss can finally happen.

- Enjoying Reward Meals in This Phase

Although maintaining weight loss is a lifelong effort, we can still have some "reward meals" in this phase. The goal is to keep to your healthy new eating habits and have two "reward meals" on the weekends. I find that as much as I enjoy my reward meals, I begin to look forward to going back to my healthy eating habits because of how they make me look and feel. By adding these reward meals on the weekends, you keep your metabolism guessing. Since your metabolism is so well trained due to healthy eating habits, two reward meals on the weekend will not have an adverse affect on your weight-loss goals. I would caution you that if you do eat a few reward meals and it causes you to revert to your old eating habits, then avoid them altogether. It's not worth losing all the success and progress that you've gained. So give yourself permission to have less-than-healthy foods for two meals per week, with the understanding that you'll spend the rest of the week eating healthy, fat burning, detoxifying foods that help keep you slim. For me, on the weekends —especially while I'm watching sports—I enjoy a thin-crust pizza and a diet soda to the fullest.

During this phase, you will reach your desired weight and begin to enjoy optimal health. This phase teaches you everything you need to know for lifetime weight control. You can expect to experience not only a lean body but also a healthy one, and a healthy body is a sexy body! You will begin to have fewer health issues and ailments and you will increase your vitality and well-being for life. You now understand which foods give your unique body the ability to stay slim, healthy, and energetic. You will continue to eat these foods and may even include a few "reward meals" on the weekend. The dietary recommendations, food choices, and supplements in the DHEMM System can help your body stay clean and lean with no further toxic buildup to hinder your weight-loss efforts.

Move (M) — Get Moving Without Going To The Gym Or "Working Out"

Most of us spend the majority of the day sitting. We ride to work in a car, bus, or subway; we sit in front of an office computer working and then we ride back home only to watch our favorite television shows seated comfortably on the sofa. For many of us, the television has become our best friend and primary source of entertainment and babysitter for our children. Our bodies suffer because we sit for fourteen or fifteen hours or more a day. It weakens our heart, slows our metabolism, and compromises our muscle strength. We used to sit when we needed a break from our hectic day, but now we sit more than 80 percent of our waking hours. The way we diet and exercise today does not work because it's unnatural. We can't just be sedentary for fifteen hours a day and think thirty minutes on the treadmill, only burning about 250 calories, is all the physical activity we need. We should be burning calories through constant physical activity throughout each day. Additionally, when we try to diet by selectively eliminating entire food groups, we often fail because we need all the foundation foods if our bodies are to stay healthy and lean. Our bodies thrive off nourishment and sustenance, not starvation and deprivation. A decade ago, there weren't half as many gyms as there are currently, and yet we didn't struggle with obesity the way we do today. A century ago, people managed their weight because they moved; they moved to find food, they moved while they worked, and they moved for recreation. The modern electronic age has made us lazier than ever. At work, we don't even walk right down the hall to talk to a coworker. Instead, we use email or text messages. Our fingers are the only body parts that might possibly be gaining muscle strength and endurance.

The DHEMM System isn't an anti-exercise program, nor am I proposing that you do not exercise. Exercise is great for your overall cardiovascular health but is not a major factor in weight loss. In this book, we discuss the real factors that produce rapid and sustained weight loss. I believe being physically active is important but that strenuous exercise—thirty to sixty minutes of aerobic exercise—is not a requirement for losing body fat. More physical activity throughout each day is what you need to eliminate excess body fat. So, the goal is simple: get moving and become more active, and you will enhance both your weight-loss efforts and your overall health. And getting moving does not necessarily mean going to the gym. In this section, we want to discuss how you burn calories throughout the day doing everyday activities, as well as tips for achieving a higher level of fitness. You burn calories while you walk from the subway to wherever you're going, while you clean the house, while you go grocery shopping, and while you dance and have fun. What we won't focus on is going to the gym or working out as the primary method for getting physically active. If you're like me, you struggle to find time to go somewhere to work out. Going to the gym to work out for an hour does not necessarily make us physically active. Being physically active involves the big and small movements we make throughout each day. It's important to note that you should continue detoxifying, eating clean and balanced foods, and using the nutritional supplements discussed in Phases 1 and 2 to serve as your lifelong plan for maintaining permanent weight loss and optimal health.

Overcoming Common Excuses for Not Being Physically Active

So what's your excuse for not being physically active? First, we want to make sure that you overcome the common excuses that many people give for not being physically active. Here are the top five excuses:

I don't have enough time: Many people lead very busy and hectic lives that begin from the moment they wake up until they lie down at night to go to sleep. This causes many people to use lack of time as the reason they are not more physically active. Many men and women in the corporate world say their work schedule is too hectic. For many women, it's work, the kids, and the household that keep them too busy to get active. However, in this section, you'll learn easy and effective ways to get more physically active without going to the gym or finding hours of time to work out. If you have committed to getting slim and healthy, then you will need to also make the commitment to incorporate physical activity into your daily life. Just think about how much time you spend watching your favorite sitcom or reality show. If you can do that, you can find time to get active. Even if you just incorporate short bursts of activity throughout the day, it will yield you very good results. As an example, when you go to the mall or grocery store, choose the parking spot farthest away from the door to ensure that you walk a few extra steps as you go about your daily routine. Just taking a ten-minute walk will clear your head and allow you to think, refocus, and get your mind right. So, instead of stressing about trying to find an hour to go to the gym, try to find ten minutes here and there to move throughout each day.

I'm too tired: This one is a catch-22 situation because if you were more physically active, you'd have more energy, but until you get more physically active, you don't have the energy to get started. During this time, it is so important to gradually get physically active so that you don't push yourself too hard. The more you move, the more your metabolism and hormonal levels will improve, allowing you to get even more active. Expect your energy levels to improve first, and then over time, you'll begin to activate and strengthen your muscles with the recommendations outlined in this book. I promise you that pressing through your fatigue will help you regain the energy you need throughout each day.

I'm embarrassed: You might be embarrassed by being overweight or obese, but if you do nothing, you'll surely remain overweight and will likely gain even more weight. Use your embarrassment as motivation to do something about it. Being overweight or out of shape sends a message that you are not taking care of your body and your health. Don't hesitate to put on big baggy clothes if you feel that you want to hide your body, but by all means, get moving. You will experience so much confidence and joy when you slim down and can begin to wear more fitted clothing. You can also get moving in the comfort of your home or while at work. Getting physically active doesn't require a trip to the gym, which can be intimidating for someone really out of shape. So, if you're embarrassed, get over it! We've all been there. It's time to let your embarrassment motivate you to create a body you can be proud to show off.

I get bored exercising: I get bored doing anything I don't want to do. That's life. But I had to begin to think of getting physically active as important to my health goals. Also, I think it is imperative that your physical activity be incorporated around your hobbies or things you enjoy.

One way to eliminate the boredom of physical activity is to engage in it with a friend, an accountability buddy who can help keep you motivated and help pass the time away. Also, variety is the spice of life, so mix it up and do different activities like walking, washing the car, yoga, gardening, etc. Keep doing different activities until you find the ones that are just right for you.

I can't afford it: It doesn't require money to get physically active. If you look at the list of activities I recommend for getting moving, you'll notice that many of them are free, easy, and actually fun. If lack of money is an issue, then know that it is a false perception that getting fit requires a gym membership. It simply does not.

Why Physical Activity Instead of Exercise?

There are many types of physical activity. Exercise is just one type of physical activity where you set aside a time to go work out or move your body. Exercise, which has some good health benefits, is when you set aside time for physical activity that increases your heart and lung activity while also strengthening your muscles and joints. However, physical activity is actually any kind of movement. It can be big or small movement, but it is anything that gets you on your feet and moving your body. Our goal is for you to be physically active throughout the day, even if you never go to the gym to exercise or work out. The good news is that even a minimal amount of physical activity goes a long way toward improving your health and meeting your weight-loss goals. Your goal is to move from being physically inactive to more physically active until your overall fitness level improves. You don't have to be a gym rat or bodybuilder to maintain a moderate or acceptable level of fitness. Being physically active keeps your blood flowing and your heart pumping and keeps your mind sharp as oxygen flows to each cell in your body. Physical activity keeps your metabolism revved up throughout the day. Additionally, your muscles allow glucose (the primary source of energy from carbohydrates) to be better utilized, which will help prevent blood sugar and insulin spikes. Physical activity has also been known to improve insulin function in the body, which is especially helpful for those who have insulin resistance. A short daily walk has even been proven to reduce the risk of developing diabetes, cancer, heart disease, high blood pressure, and many other diseases.

Using a Step Counter

A study by Dr. James Hill found that overweight people took about 1,500 to 2,000 fewer steps a day than those who maintained a healthy weight. This means that if you can find a way to get 2,000 more steps—only about four city blocks—into your day, it could help you get to your healthy weight faster. The more steps you take, the more you speed up your metabolism and burn calories and fat. This is probably why people who live in cities maintain a healthier weight, overall, than people who live in less-dense, rural areas and drive everywhere.

To determine how much physical activity you currently get, you may want to purchase a step counter, also called a pocket pedometer. The step counter will count how many steps you take in a given day. This will give you a picture of your current level of physical activity. A step counter is inexpensive and easy to use. You just clip it onto your skirt or pants in the morning and leave it on all day until you go to bed at night. Write down how many steps you take for about three days just following your normal daily routine. If you are taking 5,000 steps per day or less, you are considered relatively inactive or sedentary. Your goal should be to take 7,500 steps or more per day to be considered physically active, and, of course, the more the better. One way to accomplish this is to try to add 250 steps each week until you reach a level of 7,500 or more per day. In fact, as you begin to lose weight, you'll naturally have more energy to become more physically active each week. Of course, if your normal routine includes going to the gym, that's even better because the extra steps and movement during your workout will go toward your daily step count. The step counter keeps you motivated because it's a visual reminder to get moving throughout each day.

Tips for Getting More Physically Active

There are many great ways to get physically active without going to the gym. The goal is to make small changes in your personal and professional life that are easy to do with minimal planning and commitment. As an example, a client of mine purchased a minicycle, a set of pedals that sits on the floor or under a desk. Her goal was to use it while she sat and watched her favorite television drama. She said she kept the resistance pretty low so it wasn't too strenuous but she constantly pedaled very slowly. As a result, she lost two pounds in the first week. So she doubled the amount of time she pedaled on the minicycle while watching TV and lost three pounds the second week. It became an easy habit because she would get in a rhythm and forget she was still pedaling after a while.

Some people have gone so far as to include portable walking workstations in their office so they can either stand up or walk on a treadmill while they work or talk on the phone. You can also use the minicycle under your desk. I personally know women who have lost pounds and inches in one week just by using a minicycle while seated at their desk for an hour or two per day. If you feel uncomfortable using a portable treadmill at work, you can stand up and pace when you're on the phone and walk up and down the stairs throughout the day instead of riding the elevator. Here are twenty-five very easy ways to simply get moving without working out or going to the gym. Please identify at least five to ten of these suggestions to incorporate into your routine, starting today. These activities can help you burn anywhere from 50 calories to 500 calories.

1. Take a brisk fifteen-minute walk at lunch. For instance, you could walk to and from a restaurant that you're visiting for lunch.
2. Work in your garden; the fresh air and natural beauty are very serene and relaxing.
3. Rake the leaves.
4. Cut your grass with a walking mower.
5. Take a yoga class, especially Bikram yoga.
6. Clean out the garage.
7. Wash the floors on your hands and knees or sweep several floors.
8. Wash your car by hand.
9. Ride your bike around the neighborhood.
10. Stroller-walk your baby.
11. Park as far as you can from the grocery store or mall and walk the remaining distance.
12. Walk more briskly in the mall while shopping.
13. While watching your favorite hour-long TV show, lift hand weights or use a minicycle to help build muscle tone and strength.
14. Pace the sidelines during your child's athletic games, which may be easy to do if you're a nervous parent!

15. Take up a new sport or hobby, like tennis, skating, bowling, bike riding, line dancing, or volleyball.

16. Get off the bus or subway one stop early and walk the remaining distance.

17. Don't email coworkers who are in your building—walk to their offices instead.

18. If you play golf, go without the golf cart.

19. Walk your dog every day.

20. Take the stairs instead of the elevator.

21. Play jump rope, double dutch, hula-hoop, or Wii with the children.

22. While on a conference call, walk around during the call.

23. Sing or play a musical instrument.

24. Turn on your favorite song and dance, dance, dance!

25. Have frequent sex, which allows you to burn about 200 calories during thirty minutes of active sex . . . not a bad alternative to the gym.

Moving from Physically Active to a High Level of Fitness

As you begin to get more physically active, look to advance to more cardio fitness and strength training. One way to do so is to engage in activities such as fast walking, swimming, bike riding, jogging, Zumba, or any other type of aerobic exercise. This will increase blood flow and circulation, drop blood pressure and cholesterol levels, and allow your body to better utilize blood sugar. Additionally, you want to engage the large muscle groups by incorporating more strength training. Ladies, don't get overwhelmed by the thought of lifting weights or pumping iron. You can actually build lean muscle mass without lifting weights while still achieving better balance and bone and joint strength. There are some very simple ways to activate and strengthen the muscles that can even be done in the privacy of your home. I personally like Bikram yoga because it stretches and strengthens the muscles and increases blood flow and circulation, making it a pretty complete workout routine.

After you become more physically active, you should begin to incorporate strength training into your routine, as it is key to building muscle and losing fat. Strength training uses resistance methods like free weights, weight machines, or your own body weight to build muscle and strength. Begin gradually by spending five minutes a day flexing muscles to maintain muscle mass. Since muscle mass burns more calories than fat, trying to maintain as much muscle mass as possible is very important. To actually build muscle, you can also lift weights, which is another option. However, if you don't want to lift weights and do bodybuilding, you can help keep the muscles toned and lean by using your body weight to stress your muscles a few minutes every day.

Spending just five minutes every morning flexing your muscles reminds your brain that you need your muscles and triggers the brain to burn fat instead. Short mini-muscle activities will help with muscle toning and avoid muscle atrophy.

Each day you should take five minutes to do the following mini-muscle exercises to activate and strengthen your muscles:

- Sit-ups
- Push-ups

- Lunges and squats
- Standing heel raises or calf raises
- Dumbbell weights to lift arms in the front and sides, as well as leg squats

Get moving and get your heart pumping by doing things that are quick, enjoyable, and easy so that "exercise" becomes a natural part of your everyday life. Exercise isn't something you have to go somewhere to do. You can and should "exercise" throughout the day to keep your metabolism supercharged. Forget the "no pain, no gain" idea. It's not true. Easy, natural movements like walking will bring you significant gain as it relates to maintaining muscles, getting your heart rate up, and keeping your metabolism revved up throughout the day.

Why Whole-Body Vibration Is Effective for Weight Loss

You may not have even heard of it yet, but whole-body vibration (WBV) is the exercise of the future and could likely become as common as the treadmill is today. The WBV machine uses a vibrating plate that you stand on for ten to fifteen minutes, causing rapid muscle contractions that burn calories and provide you with muscle strength that you could otherwise get by working out for an hour in the gym. However, WBV involves no sweating or discomfort and leaves you feeling rejuvenated, calmer, and slimmer. Many of the world's best athletes in the NFL, NHL, NBA, the Olympics, as well as Hollywood celebrities, are using WBV to lose weight, build muscle tone and bone density, relieve back pain and arthritis, improve circulation, and speed up metabolism. As a woman, I've found it to be especially beneficial for burning fat and cellulite around the thighs, hips, and buttocks.

The stimulation of whole-body vibration exercise delivers quick results that are simple yet phenomenal. WBV puts the muscles in a situation where they must expand and contract continually at a rapid rate, about twenty-five to fifty times per second, which helps to strengthen them. These contractions pump extra oxygen into the cells, which allows them to repair and regenerate quickly, resulting in amazing body transformations. Keep in mind, though, that maximum fat burning and weight loss is accomplished through WBV only when combined with proper nutrition. The muscle contractions caused by a vibration plate will probably not build as much muscle mass as lifting weights, but unless you're a bodybuilder, it is still very effective for maintaining muscle tone and strength.

The results of a study that took place over a few years shocked many doctors globally. Research showed that vibration exercise was four times as effective as traditional exercise for weight loss. Additionally, the group of people who used WBV kept the weight off six months after discontinuing the use of the vibration machine. Those who only dieted or either dieted with traditional exercise all gained the weight back plus some. There are two main types of WBV machines, those that vibrate up and down using a piston-like motion (lineal) and others that vibrate from side to side like an oscillating teeter-totter (pivotal). I have personally used both, and my preference is the pivotal machines. Both machines are proven to be effective, but you should research both types if you're interested in starting a WBV routine. You can also target muscle groups by moving to different positions on the vibration machine to get even faster muscle-building results. Vibration machines are all the rage among celebrities and top athletes whose livelihood depends on their bodies being in top condition, yet they are too busy to spend hours sweating in a gym.

Here's a quick recap of what you need to do during this phase to get physically active and to reach a higher level of fitness.

• Identify your top excuses for not moving: The top five excuses as to why people don't get more physically active were discussed in this section. See if any of these excuses are holding you back, and if so, commit to overcoming them.

• Measure your current level of physical activity: To determine how much physical activity you currently get, purchase a step counter, also called a pocket pedometer, to count how many steps you take in a given day. If you don't have a step counter, just be mindful of how much you move around each day. Your goal should be to increase your movement each day so that you get more physically active week by week.

• Select at least five ways to get moving: Choose from the list of twenty-five easy ways to simply get moving without working out or going to the gym or come up with your own ideas. Incorporate your choices into your routine starting today.

• Continue detoxifying your body, eating clean and balanced foods, and taking nutritional supplements. I want to encourage you to live life the way it was meant to be lived: active, engaged, and as a full participant. Get out of your chair, get on your feet, and go live life. Since the majority of our weight and health problems can be eliminated by following the detox guidelines, clean and balanced food recommendations, and the get-moving tips outlined in the DHEMM System, you can achieve optimal health. You will enjoy your new body, energy, health, and well-being. Get excited about your new life. It is not just about weight-loss—it's a journey toward optimal health and wellness. You'll love the way your body transforms, and you'll be thrilled about your results.

Scott J. Barnard

CHAPTER 4

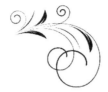

ISSUES FOR WOMEN ONLY

Research has confirmed that it is more difficult for women to lose weight than men because women's bodies are simply more efficient at storing fat. Therefore, women have to be much more deliberate about losing body fat and managing their weight. The DHEMM System allows you to make some key changes to your diet and lifestyle that help you discover a slimmer, sexier, healthier you! In this section, we'll explore some natural ways to help you achieve your most beautiful, youthful, and energetic self. We'll discuss unique issues affecting women, such as dealing with menopausal weight gain and aging skin, and provide some fun ways to get fit and sexy.

I believe that natural, healthy eating is the secret to inner and outer beauty. When you eat natural, organic foods, you simply look and feel better and younger. Once you eat in a manner that keeps your cells clean and healthy, you will begin to look radiant, despite your age. Human beings are designed to eat a diet primarily made up of fruits, vegetables, seeds, and nuts. With these types of natural, healthy foods, our bodies flourish and receive all of the necessary nutrients to keep our bodies toxin-free and looking our most beautiful. Many begin the DHEMM System to simply lose weight but they end up noticing a dramatic improvement in their health, with renewed energy and a decrease in their ailments and illnesses.

When you begin the DHEMM System, one of the first places you'll see changes is in the quality of your skin. Healthy eating and living will remove years from your face, eliminate wrinkles, fade age spots, and give you a "second youth." Your skin will become supple, and acne will clear up. Your eyes will become brighter and begin to sparkle. The dark circles and puffiness will diminish as well as the yellowness in the whites of your eyes. On the inside of your body, your cells will become rejuvenated as well, causing your organs to function more efficiently. The journey through detox fasting and cleansing is not only good for weight loss, but it is also a pathway to a second youth, greater mental clarity, and balanced moods.

Top Five Foods to Slow Aging, Fight Wrinkles, and Keep Skin Youthful

Have you noticed that your skin has begun to look dull and tired? Have you noticed a few fine lines and wrinkles? Has your youthful glow begun to fade? There are natural ways to provide your skin with the nutrients it needs to be healthier, brighter, and younger-looking! The following five foods will slow the aging of your skin and diminish the wrinkles and fine lines.

• Green leafy veggies: These foods contain vitamin A and beta-carotene and help you have bright and smooth skin. As far as food goes, it doesn't get much better than green leafy vegetables, such as kale, spinach, collards, etc. Vitamin A helps your skin produce more fresh, new cells and get rid of the old ones, reducing dryness and keeping your face looking bright and young.

• Citrus fruits: Vitamin C, a prime ingredient in tons of beauty creams, aids in the production of collagen. Once you turn thirty-five, collagen starts to break down, leaving your skin saggy. Citrus fruits, like oranges, lemons, grapefruits, and even tomatoes, contain vitamin C, and eating them helps you have smooth and tight/taut skin.

• Berries (especially blueberries and blackberries): These delicious berries keep skin looking younger longer and help fight wrinkles. Berries are considered by many experts to be one of the best food sources of antioxidants, which target free radicals that can wreak havoc on skin cells. Blueberries, in particular, are good for fighting aging, and the best are organic wild blueberries. Fresh or frozen blueberries are very good options also.

• Nuts and seeds: These foods contain vitamin E, which helps you have soft, youthful-looking skin. Incorporate more of the easily digestible seeds and nuts, like almonds, pistachios, walnuts, flaxseed, pumpkin seeds, sesame seeds, and sunflower seeds, into your diet to help provide that youthful, soft skin.

• Seafood: The omega-3 fatty acids and zinc in seafood reduce dryness and inflammation of the skin. Most of us have heard that fish can be really good for overall health—it's a primary component in what's known as the "Mediterranean diet." Many types of fish and shellfish can also work wonders for the skin, especially oysters, salmon, and tuna.

Supplements for Youthful, Glowing Skin

You can supplement your diet with certain vitamins and other ingredients that specifically support healthy, radiant hair, skin, and nails.

• Vitamin C is a natural Botox. Women with higher dosages of vitamin C in their diet were 11 percent less likely to develop wrinkles.

• Vitamin E restores moisture to the skin and slows the aging of skin cells. Green leafy vegetables and nuts are good sources of vitamin E.

• Vitamin A also helps to keep wrinkles away. The best forms of vitamin A are its derivatives, such as retinoids like Retin-A and the more moisturizing Renova. They work by removing the top layer of dead skin cells while generating collagen in the skin. Collagen is the skin's structural fiber, and as we get older, it breaks down, creating fine lines and larger pores. Skincare experts disagree on all sorts

of things, but most of them consider retinoids to be a miracle skin saver. Retinoid treatments can also help with acne, age spots, sun damage, and freckles.
• Niacin (vitamin B3) is used for a variety of skin problems, including acne, inflammation, sagging skin, and dull skin tone. Regular use of niacin will help to reduce these ailments.
• Omega-3 fatty acids are "healthy fats" that help maintain cell membranes so that they efficiently allow water and nutrients in and keep toxins out.
They also help to protect skin against sun damage. You don't necessarily have to take each of these as individual supplements. There are multivitamins targeted for healthy hair, skin, and nails that contain many of these ingredients.

Reduce Cellulite and Sagging Skin

Cellulite is the dimpled accumulation of stored fat on our thighs and buttocks caused by a sluggish lymphatic system. The lymphatic system is a secondary circulatory system underneath the skin that rids the body of toxic wastes, bacteria, and dead cells. By cleansing the liver and lymphatic system, you help rid the body of fatty deposits—the key to diminishing cellulite. Another cause of cellulite is loose or weakening skin and connective tissues that are unable to keep the fat tissues contained within their compartments. As the fat tissues or deposits escape through weakened connective strands, they create the dimply, pebbly effect known as cellulite. So strengthening the skin and muscles is a great preventive measure for cellulite. Foods containing protein help to firm up muscles that can keep fat stores in place and reduce the dimpled effect of cellulite.

Here are some specific tips for reducing cellulite:
• Body brushing. Body brushing improves circulation, removes dead skin layers, and encourages cell renewal for a much smoother-textured skin. This process also eliminates toxins by stimulating the lymphatic system.
• Drink green tea: Green tea burns fat really well, especially stubborn fat areas like cellulite. I try to drink two cups per day.
• Eating lean proteins: When your body lacks protein, your facial skin, and the skin on your arms and legs, begins to sag due to lost collagen. Those with thinning hair and too many wrinkles for their age, or puffy eyes, may lack protein. Your muscles, hair, nails, skin, and eyes are made of protein. It is necessary for tissue repair, and every cell in our body needs protein to maintain its life and replace dead cells. If you follow the guidelines in this book (i.e., the amount of protein to eat) daily, you will get the sufficient amount that your body needs every day. However, if you are very active or weightlifting, then you should increase your protein intake, typically done by drinking protein powder shakes, to repair and rebuild muscle.

Reduce Belly Fat for a Sexy Waistline

There are some unique challenges we women face when it comes to losing weight. One of the questions most commonly asked of me is, "How do I get rid of belly fat?" Let's discuss belly fat in general and then discuss the following strategies for achieving a slimmer waistline:

- Get rid of toxins
- Eliminate stress
- Treat estrogen dominance

If we look at people with flat stomachs and six-packs, they look like a picture of good health, fitness, and strength. A flat, tight stomach is a sign that someone is in control of her body and in control of her health. Most people will admit to wanting a thinner waistline, and this is not shallow at all. Tight, sexy abs are rated the sexiest body part by many men and women. When you appear in control of your health, it's a sign to the world that you are not only a highly motivated, disciplined, and healthy person, but that you are an attractive and desirable mate as well. We all know what belly fat is; we see it every day when we walk out of the house. Belly fat, known as visceral fat, is located behind your abdominal wall and surrounds your internal organs. Visceral fat typically shows as the belly fat/spare tire around the waist and midsection. Even thin people can begin to store excess weight around the stomach and midsection. Visceral fat contains toxins and substances that are harmful to our health and can affect the nervous system and the endocrine (hormonal) system, which ends up affecting metabolism and appetite.

Most people do not know that belly fat is the most dangerous fat on the body. Because of where it's located around the delicate organs, it has the potential to destroy good health, or worse yet, kill you. Because belly fat resides within striking distance of your heart, liver, and other organs, it is to blame for many health conditions. According to a 2006 study published in the journal Obesity, visceral fat is a significant predictor of early death. In other words, visceral fat means you have an increased risk for a shortened life. Even if you removed visceral fat via liposuction, it may cause you to look physically better, but it does little for improving your health because the dangers of visceral fat would still exist for you. The good news is that even a minimal amount of physical activity and dietary changes will go a long way in shrinking visceral fat.

Get Rid of Toxins to Decrease Belly Fat

Studies have shown that exposing yourself to an excessive amount of environmental toxins increases belly fat. Thus, a very effective way to address this visceral fat/belly fat is to eliminate toxins from the body.

Eliminate Stress to Reduce Belly Fat

Stress may be another factor that affects belly fat. When you are stressed, your body releases a hormone called cortisol (also known as stress hormone). Studies have shown that when cortisol is released into the bloodstream, you become less sensitive to leptin, the hormone that tells your brain you are full. When this happens, you tend to eat more and more and begin to crave sugar. And fat caused by stress tends to get stored in the belly. To reduce the stress in your life, follow these tips:

• Place "happy photos" at work and in your car (like on the visor). When you look at them, they will immediately take you to a happy place, causing stress levels to decrease.

• Make love: The more we make love, the more endorphins our brains release. These "neurohormones" act as natural painkillers and help to alleviate anxiety.

• Schedule "playtime" with your significant other or children. Doing fun things like miniature golf, bowling, and seeing a movie can take your mind off your stress.

• Smile often and laugh a lot: If you have a favorite comedian, include a CD in your car to listen to as you drive to and from work. Or watch movies that make you laugh out loud. Or listen to music that calms you down or makes you sing along.

• Get a massage: Deep-pressure massage stimulates the nerves that cause levels of the stress hormone cortisol to diminish. Research has also shown that those who give massages reduce their own levels of stress hormones.

• Get moving: It is well documented that regular physical activity or exercise helps to alleviate stress and raise body temperature, which helps the body prepare for sleep. There's strong evidence that moderate exercise like brisk walking activates the "feel-good" neurotransmitters dopamine and serotonin, which reduce the symptoms of depression.

• Build better relationships: The biggest enemy of good health is stress. The biggest enemy of stress is solid relationships with other people. So show more respect and compassion to other people, even more than you feel they deserve. This might seem to hurt you in the short term, but it is a sure investment in the long term.

• Sleep more: Too many Americans are sleep-deprived. However, I can honestly say I am not one of them. I am a huge fan of sleep. I get my eight hours of sleep every night, and if I fall short one night, I make up for it over the weekend. Sleep is the body's way of recharging the system and is the easiest yet most underrated activity to heal the body. Sleep also helps to eliminate puffy red eyes and dark circles. There isn't anything that can compensate for lack of sleep. Lack of sleep accelerates wear and tear, accelerating aging, and pushes the body out of its natural balance and rhythm. Shortchanging sleep time or going to bed stressed interferes with the best time for losing those extra pounds. So be sure to relax or meditate before going to sleep. Relaxing causes cortisol levels to drop, which will in turn help your body burn more calories. In short, getting enough sleep helps you burn more calories at night and during the day.

If you are like me and have been frustrated with extra fat and bloating around your waist and abdomen, you will also be pleased to know that sometimes those extra pounds have little to do with how many crunches you're doing or how much less food you're eating and everything to do with a shift in hormones that happens with almost everyone over the age of thirty-five. Excess belly fat is often due to a hormonal imbalance called estrogen dominance, which can occur primarily in women but sometimes in men also. If you don't address estrogen dominance, your stubborn belly fat will likely remain and be impossible to lose no matter how much you cut down on calories or work out. The good news is that estrogen dominance can be treated, and once your hormones have been properly balanced, the extra fat around your waist will begin to melt away.

In women, and oftentimes men, higher estrogen levels cause the body to store fat around the waist and abdomen area. More specifically, in women, estrogen dominance causes fat to be stored around the stomach, waist, hips, and thighs, causing us to look round or pear-shaped once we get in our forties. For men, it causes them to have the fat belly that looks like a spare tire around their waist. The three best ways to address belly fat caused by estrogen dominance are:

• Eating a clean and balanced diet. This will ensure that you avoid foods that cause estrogen-mimicking toxins to circulate in the body.

• Using natural hormone replacement therapy, also called bio identical hormone replacement therapy (BHRT), to restore hormonal balance.

• Taking nutritional supplements that eliminate excess estrogen circulating in the body, thereby providing the hormonal balance required to lose unwanted fat, namely belly fat.

Women who address these three factors successfully relieve their symptoms of estrogen dominance, namely that bloated belly, within one to two months. For me personally, to have my stomach literally deflate from bloated to flat happened within a few short weeks. Most women over forty begin to experience some of the trouble areas we've discussed in this section: belly fat, cellulite, and fine lines and wrinkles. Now you have some real strategies to deal with the trouble spots and reverse the aging process so that you will look and feel more youthful.

Stop Weight Gain During Perimenopause And Menopause

If you're over thirty-five, you may have begun to notice a few extra pounds around your waist, hips, thighs, and butt. You may not have changed your eating habits or exercise routine but may still be unable to maintain your weight. You should be happy to know that you are definitely not alone. Weight gain, along with overall change in body shape, is normal and should be expected. Over 90 percent of women gain weight between the ages of thirty-five and fifty-five. The average weight gain during this period of perimenopause and menopause is fifteen to twenty pounds, around one to two pounds per year, and the earlier you move into perimenopause the more extreme and rapid the weight gain will be. It's not just that you gain weight, it's also how the weight tends to be distributed around your waistline, belly, thighs, hips, and butt area that makes your body appear to be more round and less curvy. As your estrogen levels decline, they also affect the production of collagen, which results in drier, thinner skin, saggy tissue, and lack of muscle tone—all factors that contribute to a change in your body shape.

Even if you eat in the same manner as you did for years, you can expect weight gain as you get closer to the perimenopause/menopause years. Weight gain, especially around the midsection, as well as soft, jiggly arms, hips, and thighs, are all unfortunate realities of getting older. I have personally experienced this frustration and know many other women who have experienced this undesirable weight gain. Unfortunately, our bodies become naturally insulin-resistant as we age, which makes us more inclined to store fat, especially around the waist. Additionally, our ovaries are beginning to produce less estrogen during perimenopause, which causes the body's fat cells to try to produce more estrogen. While fat cells are not the primary source of estrogen production in the body, they do produce estrogen. However, once you achieve hormonal balance, you can get back to a body that burns fat instead of storing it.

Weight gain in this stage of life is due to fluctuating hormones, but the good news is that you can achieve a better hormone balance. You do not have to accept getting heavier and heavier as you age, and yes, you can lose those extra pounds.

Understanding Perimenopause and Menopause

Menopause is the time in a woman's life when her menstruation stops and she is no longer fertile (i.e., no longer able to become pregnant). Perimenopause is the stage that precedes menopause, and it may last for many years. It's the transition from normal menstrual periods to no periods at all. Perimenopausal women can be emotional, moody, and irritable because they are still getting a period, albeit it is very irregular—sometimes heavy and sometimes very light. This rather severe state of hormonal imbalance causes hormonal surges and symptoms. This stage officially marks the beginning of hormonal decline, resulting in symptoms such as weight gain, mood swings, hot flashes, sleeplessness, lack of sex drive, fatigue, and irritability. Women in their late thirties and early forties may already be beginning this transition, and as their bodies experience hormonal confusion, unexplained symptoms begin to pop up. (When I went through it, I got seasonal allergies for the first time in my life.)

Even though perimenopause and menopause are normal processes that all women will go through the symptoms associated with them can be minimized or avoided altogether. If you are in this stage of life, you have to be diligent about finding the right doctor who will understand what is really going on in your body. Most doctors will simply treat the symptoms; very few tie all of them together and address the root cause of the problem. The underlying problem is hormone loss, and the sooner you replace these hormones, the better you will look and feel. No one is going to be as committed to doing this as you. Know that perimenopause is your wake-up call to take action to restore your health back to a state where you felt balanced, youthful, and energetic.

By the time you get to menopause, you should already be so actively balancing your hormones that this next transition in life should not have to feel painful and depressing, and you should experience fewer symptoms of hot flashes, night sweats, mood swings, and other menopausal symptoms. You will begin even more hormonal decline, but you'll also be able to continue tweaking your hormones so you feel balanced and healthy. It's important to research and understand what happens with hormonal decline in each transition phase of your life, from perimenopause to menopause and beyond.

Three Key Sex Hormones That Affect Weight Gain

There are three key sex hormones that can become imbalanced as you age. Fluctuating hormonal levels of estrogen, progesterone, and testosterone cause weight gain, mood swings, irregular menstrual cycles, and many other symptoms that we'll discuss in this section.

- Estrogen

Estrogen, produced by the ovaries, is what transforms us from girls into women. It gives us our curves and helps regulate our passage through fertility and menstruation. Estrogen occurs in the body in three compounds: estradiol (most potent estrogen), estrone (dominant estrogen after menopause), and estriol (weakest form of estrogen, at its highest levels during pregnancy). Estrogen stimulates growth in breasts, ovaries, and the uterus. Both men and women have estrogen, but women have much higher levels of it. Estrogen is one of the two main hormones produced in the ovaries. The other, progesterone, is produced primarily in the second half of a woman's menstrual cycle. When women reach their thirties and forties, it is very common for the balance between the two hormones to shift heavily toward estrogen, causing a condition known as estrogen dominance, resulting in night sweats, depression, fatigue, weight gain, anxiety, blood sugar imbalance, low sex drive, dry skin and hair, cellulite, and brain fog. Too much estrogen in the body also causes salt and water retention, making us look bloated, flabby, and soft. However, the estrogen and progesterone levels can be balanced to relieve these symptoms.

- Progesterone

Your body secretes progesterone every month after an egg is released. During times of high levels of progesterone, the body burns 100 to 300 more calories per day than it does during times of high levels of estrogen. Progesterone also helps to reduce bloating and uterine fibroids, improves libido, and boosts mental clarity. As I stated earlier, when your progesterone levels overall start to drop, estrogen dominance sets in, and you may experience early symptoms of menopause, known as perimenopause. When you have low levels of progesterone, you may also experience premenstrual syndrome and possibly depression. The sudden appearance of abdominal fat, in particular, is a sign that the body's internal hormonal ratio of progesterone to estrogen is unbalanced. A primary goal of hormone balancing is to restore the balance between estrogen and progesterone to create harmony and balance in our body. When estrogen and progesterone are properly balanced, these two hormones help the body burn fat, boost metabolism, and relieve the symptoms of estrogen dominance.

Luckily, there are foods that enhance your progesterone levels, allowing you to better metabolize fat and sleep better. The B vitamin family, in particular B6, is key to enhancing progesterone levels. You can get B vitamins in meat, poultry, fish, beans, and some fruits and vegetables, like bananas, avocados, spinach, and tomatoes. Another key nutrient that will help progesterone production is magnesium, found in dark green leafy vegetables, eggs, meat, seeds, nuts, and beans. Fortunately, these foods high in magnesium will also keep your liver healthy. Poor liver function causes hormonal imbalances, and in particular, suppresses progesterone.

- Testosterone

Testosterone often is overlooked when women are dealing with perimenopause and menopausal symptoms. However, women with low testosterone levels experience fatigue, weakness, low energy, low motivation, muscle atrophy, and a lowered sex drive. Men naturally make 50 percent more testosterone than women; however, it is a vital hormone in women also. Many women are surprised to hear that testosterone is actually produced in small amounts by the ovaries and the adrenal glands. This hormone supports a woman's body by helping it to maintain its energy levels, muscle tone, vaginal elasticity, sex drive, and overall vitality.

Between the ages of thirty-five and fifty-five, women typically lose about 50 percent of their testosterone, and this too contributes to unpleasant symptoms. During perimenopause, which can begin as early as thirty-five, ovulation becomes irregular, and both progesterone and testosterone levels begin to decline. In some situations, a woman may have high levels of testosterone; when this occurs, she can experience acne or other skin breakouts, the growth of facial hair, and weight gain. As we age, we all experience a decline in hormone levels. Women lose 30 percent of their estrogen by age fifty, 75 percent of their progesterone, and 50 percent of their testosterone between ages thirty-five and fifty. Both progesterone and estrogen then continue to decline sharply after menopause. The reality is that we all experience the symptoms of hormonal decline. However, there are some ways that we can maintain a better hormonal balance and minimize these unpleasant symptoms.

When estrogen levels remain high in the body relative to progesterone, the result is a condition known as estrogen dominance. The primary symptoms of estrogen dominance are weight gain (especially around the abdomen, hips, and thighs), sluggish metabolism, mood swings, irregular periods, and bloating. I know estrogen dominance all too well, and every one of these symptoms was very real and very frustrating to me. Estrogen dominance also causes increased bloating and water retention— which may not be the result of more fat but still makes you look heavier and causes your blood sugar to fluctuate, which increases your appetite and slows your metabolism. When women are menstruating, this bloating occurs right around the menstrual cycle. When women no longer have periods and are not producing progesterone, the bloating will be a constant problem. Progesterone acts as a natural diuretic. Progesterone also encourages the body to use calories from food for energy; without enough progesterone, the body is compromised in its ability to metabolize calories, and the calories get stored as fat in the body.

Estrogen dominance can cause insulin resistance, which causes insulin to be released more often than itnis needed. This extra release of insulin causes the body to crave sugar and to store fat. However, balancing estrogen and progesterone levels helps to regulate the release of insulin. In both sexes, estrogen dominance is thought to be one of the leading causes of breast, uterine, and prostate cancers. Contrary to the popular belief that estrogen is a "female" hormone, men can also be estrogen dominant. One possible cause of estrogen dominance is exposure to environmental estrogens, and men are exposed to the same ones as women. Men who show signs of estrogen dominance are typically over the age of forty and experience weight gain around the middle, hair loss, development of breasts, and fatigue. The "thickening" of women's bodies and the "softening" of men's bodies are often related to excess estrogen. When in excess, estrogen promotes the growth of estrogen-sensitive tissues, known as "stubborn fat" because they are highly resistant to fat burning. Even if you eat less and exercise, this doesn't help remove the estrogen-sensitive fat. You get caught in a vicious cycle as excess estrogen promotes fat gain; the enlarged estrogen-sensitive fat tissue produces more estrogen within its cells, which then promotes more fat gain, and so on.

Common symptoms of estrogen dominance include:
- Stubborn fat/weight gain around stomach area, hips, thighs, and butt
- Water retention/bloating
- Tender breasts
- Low libido
- Problematic PMS/menstrual cramps
- Dry skin/vaginal dryness
- Mood swings or irritability
- Hot flashes/night sweats
- Insomnia
- Brain fog or "fuzzy thinking"
- Irregular periods or heavy or long-lasting periods
- Fatigue
- Depression or low motivation
- Cyclical migraine headaches
- Infertility or frequent miscarriage
- Fibrocystic breasts
- Uterine fibroids
- Endometriosis
- Low-thyroid symptoms
- Polycystic ovary syndrome (PCOS)
- Breast cancer

Bioidentical Hormone Replacement Therapy (BHRT) to Naturally Balance Hormones

The good news is that bioidentical hormone replacement therapy (BHRT) can solve the problem of estrogen dominance by allowing you to increase the amount of progesterone in your body. The result will be a reduction in or the elimination of many of the symptoms of perimenopause/menopause. But since BHRT is not very widely accepted by the medical establishment and is considered "alternative medicine," you will have to do some research to find a good doctor qualified to prescribe it. Believe me, it is well worth the search. Bioidentical hormones are hormones derived from plants, usually soybeans or wild yams, through a biochemical process that ensures that the molecular structure is identical to the hormones women make in their bodies. Synthetic hormones are not identical in either structure or activity to the natural hormones they emulate.

The body can't distinguish bioidentical hormones from the ones your ovaries produce, so they fit perfectly into the hormone receptors like a lock and key. Hormones work like a key in a lock.

Bioidentical hormones fit that lock perfectly. Synthetic hormones fit some, but not all, of the hormone receptor (lock) sites. This causes synthetic hormones to have more side effects than bioidentical hormones because of a poor lock and key fit. Bioidentical hormones (key) fit perfectly into the hormone receptors (lock), causing the body to recognize and accept bioidentical hormones just as it would recognize and accept naturally occurring human hormones, making it both effective and safe. The great appeal of bioidentical hormones is that our bodies can metabolize them as they were designed to do, minimizing side effects. Synthetic hormones are quite strong and often produce intolerable side effects. The other important factor is that bioidentical hormones can be matched individually to each woman's hormonal needs, something that's close to impossible to do with mass-produced synthetic products. According to a study published in the Journal of the American Medical Association, synthetic hormones were found to increase a woman's risk of breast cancer, heart disease, blood clots, and stroke. Studies show that bioidentical hormones are both safer and more effective.

By adding natural, bioidentical hormones into your body, you can restore a good hormonal balance between estrogen and progesterone. Bioidentical hormones can be any of the steroid hormones, including estrogen, progesterone, or testosterone. However, many articles and blogs confuse people, making them think that natural or bioidentical hormones are the same as synthetic hormones. They are most definitely not. However, when I say bioidentical progesterone, I mean natural progesterone and not synthetic progesterone. Using a natural or bioidentical progesterone is an important factor in correcting your underlying condition of estrogen dominance, resulting in loss of those unwanted pounds. By boosting your body's progesterone levels, you can offset the excess estrogen and create a proper hormonal balance that will allow your body to burn fat more efficiently.

So, Why Don't More Physicians Know About and Prescribe Bioidentical Hormones?

The molecular structure of natural human hormones cannot be patented and neither can the identical molecular structure of bioidentical hormones. Without a patent, pharmaceutical companies cannot mass-produce, market, and sell them. No chance for big profits translates into no interest on the part of large pharmaceutical companies. Instead of selling the more natural products, pharmaceutical companies produce synthetic hormones, which are patentable because they have a slightly different molecular structure from both natural human hormones and bioidentical hormones. These companies then spend millions of dollars marketing synthetic hormones to physicians (via office presentations, forums, and meetings) so that physicians will prescribe synthetic hormones rather than bioidentical ones. The companies make billions of dollars selling these synthetic hormones.

Despite numerous credible clinical trials and research studies that validate the safety and efficacy of bioidentical hormone therapies, many doctors remain unaware of their health benefits. This may be because many doctors feel that synthetic or prescription medicines in general are the best approach to addressing symptoms. However, many practitioners who study alternative medicine focus on healing the body, not just treating symptoms. Thus, they seek out the most effective natural methods for healing the body. This is my approach, of course. Others believe that many of the universities and establishments that publish information on bioidentical hormones don't have the budgets to educate and market to doctors, who are then slow to learn of their health benefits.

How Bioidentical Hormones Help in the Battle of the Bulge

By using bioidentical progesterone, you increase your progesterone levels to neutralize estrogen dominance. The proper balance between estrogen and progesterone will help your body efficiently metabolize food so that it is not stored as fat. Additionally, progesterone acts as a natural diuretic, reducing bloating and water weight. For those who are insulin resistant, you'll be glad to know that a better balance between progesterone and estrogen slows the rapid release of insulin, thereby decreasing fat storage in the body. There are also studies that show that bioidentical progesterone can reduce estrogen's ability to stimulate cell growth that can result in cancer, thereby providing additional protection against cancer. For younger, menstruating women, bioidentical progesterone is even used to help alleviate PMS symptoms.

How to Take Bioidentical Progesterone

Bioidentical progesterone can be taken as a cream, pill, capsule, or suppository. However, topical creams have been shown to be the most effective way of taking it. If you take pills, you have to take a higher dosage because when the pill is digested, it must go through the liver to be metabolized, leaving much of the active ingredients to be excreted in the feces. So, only some of the active ingredient makes its way into the bloodstream to be used by the body. When you rub the cream form of it into your skin, it is absorbed directly into the bloodstream. Once it's in the bloodstream, the bioidentical progesterone can travel to the hormone receptor sites to be used by the body in the same manner human hormones would. As a result, a lower dosage is required when the bioidentical hormone topical cream is used. The greatest success with bioidentical hormone replacement therapy occurs when you have the help of a trained healthcare provider who can provide an individual approach to address your hormonal imbalances. You should describe every symptom you experience while using bioidentical hormones, so that your healthcare provider can tweak the dosage of hormones until you reach a balanced hormonal state. The provider should begin with laboratory tests of hormone levels (sometimes called "hormone panel") to understand your current hormone levels. The two most common types of hormone testing are saliva testing and blood testing. The correct prescription dosage, which is filled at a compounding pharmacy, will include customized bioidentical hormones based upon your hormone levels. The doctor will then monitor you monthly to ensure that your symptoms are being alleviated. Follow-up hormone tests can also be conducted in four to six months to ensure hormonal balance is restored.

If you have difficulty finding a doctor who specializes in bioidentical hormones, check your local compounding pharmacy, as it may be able to recommend doctors with this specialization. Compounding pharmacies are where doctors in your area will call to fill your custom compound of bioidentical hormone prescriptions that are prepared just for you based upon your individual needs. You can do a Google search to find local compounding pharmacies in your area or a doctor specializing in bioidentical hormone therapy. Your healthcare provider should advise you on the most efficient method for taking progesterone. However, bioidentical progesterone cream is readily available without a prescription at most health food stores and health websites. Some women who opt to begin taking over-the-counter bioidentical hormones should be aware that some over-the-counter progesterone creams are better than others. Unfortunately, there is no regulatory body that oversees the production or standardization of natural health products.

Supplements That Support Hormone Balance

When dealing with the most common form of hormonal imbalance, estrogen dominance, the most effective supplements are those that help eliminate excess estrogen from the body or metabolize estrogen so that more of the "good estrogen" is used by the body and more of the "bad estrogen" is eliminated from the body. The select group of supplements below has been proven to create hormone balance, resulting in weight loss and fewer mood swings, hot flashes, and other symptoms caused by hormonal imbalance. You should work with your healthcare provider to determine if any of these supplements would be beneficial to you.

- Calcium D-Glucarate

Calcium D-glucarate is a common nutrient found in many fruits and vegetables. This nutrient is believed to aid the body in the elimination of many harmful toxins and also lowers abnormally high levels of hormones, namely estrogen. Calcium D-glucarate inhibits the reabsorption of estrogenmimicking toxins into the bloodstream, allowing them to be excreted from the body. Women dealing with estrogen dominance can typically take 1,000 mg of calcium D-glucarate two times per day.

- Dehydroepiandrosterone (DHEA)

Dehydroepiandrosterone (DHEA) is a steroid hormone produced by the body's adrenal glands. DHEA functions as a precursor to testosterone, the male sex hormone, and estrogen, the female sex hormone. In most people, DHEA production gradually declines with age, and it is believed that supplementing our bodies' falling levels of this hormone might help turn back the hands of time and boost the body's ability to burn fat. DHEA causes weight loss through a process called thermogenesis, which is the creation of heat at a cellular level. The more thermogenesis, the higher the metabolic rate, and the more fat burned. It is recommended that you take 100 mg of DHEA daily.

- Diindolylmethane (DIM)

Diindolylmethane (DIM) is a phytonutrient, a plant compound similar to those found in cruciferous vegetables, such as broccoli, cabbage, Brussels sprouts, and cauliflower. Since it would be difficult to get enough of these vegetables through our diet daily (it would require eating two pounds of broccoli per day) to properly eliminate the bad estrogen, we can take a nutritional supplement known as DIM (diindolylmethane) to get the adequate amounts to restore hormonal balance and eliminate the symptoms of estrogen dominance. DIM eliminates excess estrogen by shifting the way estrogen is metabolized in the body. DIM allows for more of the "good estrogen" metabolites and elimination of the "bad estrogen" metabolites. DIM will not directly decrease the estrogen levels in the body, but rather will redirect how it is metabolized so that more of the "bad estrogen" metabolites are eliminated. Consuming vegetables containing DIM or a DIM supplement can help prevent the development of certain cancers. DIM has also been proven to destroy and prevent the mutation of cancer cells. DIM is believed to help prevent breast and prostate cancer by promoting a balance of good vs. bad estrogen in the body. Using a bioidentical progesterone cream in combination with DIM has been shown to even more effectively alleviate symptoms of estrogen dominance than just using the cream alone. One reason for this is that there's no ideal way to tell how much progesterone you're actually getting through the cream or how much your body is able to use, and taking the time to monitor symptoms and test for progesterone levels periodically makes the treatment a little bit slow. So the use of DIM, along with a bioidentical progesterone cream, alleviates symptoms faster.

Many practitioners recommend taking about 200 to 300 mg of DIM per day (or about 100 to 150 mg twice per day). Since it is difficult to absorb, be sure it is in the form of a specialized complex to improve bioavailability. You don't want to take plain DIM without the bioavailable complex. There are very few reported side effects from taking supplemental DIM. However, some individuals have experienced headaches, upset stomach, and gas. If this occurs, be sure to take DIM with food and to reduce the dosage and slowly work your way up to the recommended dosage.

Tips for Preventing Weight Gain During Perimenopause and Menopause

In addition to exploring BHRT and taking nutritional supplements, eating right and staying physically active will help you maintain your ideal body weight during the perimenopause and menopause phases of life. All of the advice provided in the DHEMM System is especially helpful for women in perimenopause and menopause. There are eight rules you can follow that will help you prevent weight gain during perimenopause/menopause. They are the following:

1. Maintain healthy liver function and regular bowel movements to eliminate excess estrogen from the body.

2. Avoid alcohol: It spurs the production of harmful estrogen. In fact, even one glass of alcohol a day can raise estrogen levels.

3. Minimize exposure to xenoestrogens: These are environmental chemicals in pesticides, plastics, some cosmetics, and household cleaning products that can get into your bloodstream and increase estrogen levels.

4. Eliminate sugar and starch from your diet: Get sugar out of your diet if you want to lose body fat. By sugar, I mean candy and sweets, of course, but really any starchy, processed foods that cause insulin spikes resulting in excess fat in the body. If you want to reduce fatigue and weight (fat) gain, try to have no more than two servings of starchy carbohydrates— such as potatoes and corn—per day and avoid sugary sweets altogether.

5. Eat more fiber: Fiber from whole grains, fruits, and vegetables helps to move estrogen out of the body, which helps prevent it from building up and creating a hormonal burden on your system.

6. Eat lean proteins: I discussed the value of lean protein earlier, but it really helps to offset the symptoms of perimenopause and menopause by helping maintain muscle mass, which burns more calories than fat. Whenever your body is not getting enough protein, you will begin to feel moody, emotional, anxious, and just plain tired. Good choices of protein are eggs, fish, lean beef, turkey, or chicken.

7. Eat more detoxifying foods: Add plenty of detoxifying foods to your diet, including broccoli, cauliflower, Brussels sprouts, kale, cabbage, beets, carrots, apples, ginger, onions, and celery. Eat at least five servings of fresh fruits and veggies per day. In particular, dark leafy green veggies, such as spinach, collards, and kale, are ideal. Regarding fruit, the brighter and deeper the color the better; great choices are oranges, blackberries, and apples.

8. Get moving: The unpleasant reality is that women begin to naturally lose muscle mass during middle age. So not only are we gaining and storing fat, we're losing lean muscle mass as well. This is a double whammy. So you will want to begin some physical activity to help maintain lean muscle mass as you age to boost your metabolism. At the time of this writing, I am in my forties and in perimenopause. I experienced many unpleasant symptoms of estrogen dominance, including acne, bloating, depression, hot flashes, heavy or painful periods, irregular periods, irritability, loss of muscle mass, mood swings, poor concentration, sleep disturbances, urinary incontinence, and, my least favorite, rapid unexplained weight gain. My rapid weight gain was actually alarming due to how healthy my lifestyle and eating habits were at the time.

I did my research and embraced bioidentical hormone replacement therapy and other nutritional supplements and herbs. Now, I have no problem with aging. I love being in my forties as long as I have a healthy, youthful, and energetic body. Balanced hormones bring joy, strength, and great physical and emotional health. I've learned from experience that a healthy woman is hormonally balanced. If you are frustrated with belly fat, a pear-shaped body, or bloating and water retention, the use of bioidentical hormones and other key supplements can help you restore the hormone balance and metabolic function in the body. Fat distribution will normalize, and you will begin to see the weight melt away.

Don't Like To Exercise? Try Sexercise!

Sexercising routines not only help you get fit, they also help you get your sexy back. Keep in mind that men are very visual creatures, and having a little sex appeal will not only give you more confidence in your feminine self but will also help you attract more men. There are four popular types of sexercises: pole dancing, belly dancing, Zumba, and striptease.

Pole Dancing

Although pole dancing is fast becoming a widely accepted fitness activity, there are still a lot of misconceptions about what it really is all about. Pole dancing allows many women to improve their confidence and self-esteem while becoming more fit and toned. If you get past the stigma that comes along with pole dancing, you'll find that it is a great way to build incredible strength while having loads of fun. The pole requires significant arm strength because most of the time you are using your arms to lift your entire body. There is a wide variety of exercises you can do on your pole to increase flexibility and muscle tone while performing sexy, strength-building dance moves.

Although pole dancing is associated with strippers, there's no nudity at a pole-dancing class nor are there men gawking at you during the class session. You will find women of all ages and sizes prancing around the pole, flying in the air, and spinning forward and backward, with pauses for little playful teases. Throughout the class session, students learn different pole exercise moves and eventually work their way up to performing a complete routine. Many take their newfound skills and offer their boyfriend or husband a special treat. Some join to get fit, embrace their sexuality, or simply to gain more self-confidence. Whatever the reason they join, they typically leave feeling sexy, sensual, and confident about their bodies. Pole-dancing fitness can liberate your sensuality and give you confidence in showing off your new feminine body.

Belly Dancing

Belly dancing is not only fun but is also a great form of exercise. It tones the arms, strengthens and tightens the abs and obliques, and improves flexibility. It can burn as many calories as jogging, swimming, or riding a bike but is less strenuous on the body than weight lifting and more entertaining than sitting on a bike at the gym. Belly dancing is a very different form of exercise than what you may be used to, as it is a beautiful and sensual dance form. What makes belly dancing unique is that it is a cultural experience; you learn about its Middle Eastern origins while burning fat, improving flexibility and posture, and enhancing your sexuality and femininity. Belly dancing is great for women who want sexy abs, as it's a perfect workout for your midsection, waist, and core. Belly dancing adds a whole different dimension to your fitness experience.

Zumba

Zumba is a type of fitness class that has garnered quite a bit of attention recently. A great way to firm, tone, and sweat while doing a lively, upbeat Latin dance, Zumba incorporates aerobic interval training with Latin-style dance movements to provide a refreshing change from traditional aerobics routines. Many are enamored with Zumba's many benefits for burning fat, toning muscles, and having fun. Zumba classes, which usually last about an hour, can burn up to 500 calories and really rev up your metabolism. It's a fun workout that is more of a good time than an exercise class. The dance moves are easy to learn. Instructors teach the basic routines and then add more intricate dance moves. The movements used in Zumba— such as salsa, merengue, cha-cha, mambo, and Zumba shuffle steps—all help to tone muscles. Zumba feels more like an evening at a Latin dance club than an exercise routine and is growing in popularity each day.

Striptease

Striptease is more of a seductive dance routine, typically performed in stilettos. When I attended striptease class, the dips and gyrating leg movements really helped to tone up my thighs and legs. Both striptease and pole-dance classes are great ways to embrace your sexuality and simply look and feel sexy and desirable. There are also workout videos, like Flirty Girl Fitness DVDs, if you want to work out at home as opposed to going to a dance studio. Striptease is an exercise routine that you may prefer to practice in the privacy of your own home. This will allow you to let go of your inhibitions. The more you practice, the more you'll get comfortable freeing your sensual self. The good news is that you really begin to work your muscles by gyrating and bending to the music of your choice. Once you get comfortable with your striptease routine, you may want to show it to your significant other. I'm sure he will enjoy your lean and toned body, along with your sensuality. When you get confident in your body, your movements will be beautiful and sensual, and you'll walk around the room with a wonderful, sexual presence that you and your mate will both appreciate.

Why Black Women Gain More Weight Than Other Women

The statistics are widely published. The National Center for Health Statistics reports that more than one half (54.3 percent) of Americans are obese, with black women comprising the most overweight segment of the U.S. population, followed by Hispanic women. The statistics indicate that 78 percent of us are overweight—that's nearly four out of five black women— and 54 percent of us are obese. African American women are suffering from obesity at an alarmingly disproportionate rate compared to women of other races. As I've said earlier, being overweight or obese is not always a matter of eating too much or not exercising, but this gets even more complicated for black women. There are a variety of reasons that black women are overweight or obese. I will discuss five of them in this section.

Black Woman Have a Slower Metabolism

Genetically, African American women tend to have a slower metabolism, according to research published in the American Journal of Clinical Nutrition. A University of Pennsylvania Medical Center study found that black women have "a biological disadvantage" that makes it more difficult to lose weight. Researchers have found that even at rest, overweight black women burn nearly 100 fewer calories daily compared to their overweight white peers. While this news may seem like gloom and doom for black women who want to lose weight, know that it is a challenge that can be overcome. The healthy eating and lifestyle strategies described in this book, specifically the ways to speed up your metabolism, will help you burn more calories.

Black Women Are More Prone to Insulin Resistance, Which Causes Excess Fat Storage in the Body

Black women, even if their weight is normal, may be at increased risk for insulin resistance, a condition linked to diabetes and high blood pressure, according to research by Wake Forest University School of Medicine. Insulin resistance means the body can't effectively use the hormone insulin to process glucose, forcing the pancreas to produce more insulin, and elevated insulin levels lead to excess fat storage in the body. Almost half of lean black women had insulin resistance, which was double the rate in both Hispanic and Caucasian women. The study showed that 47 percent of black women of normal weight had insulin resistance compared to less than 20 percent of the Hispanic or Caucasian women. The researchers looked at how obesity relates to insulin resistance in black, Caucasian, and Hispanic women as a part of the Insulin Resistance Atherosclerosis Study (IRAS). The research suggested that race, in addition to obesity, is an important contributor to the development of insulin resistance and type 2 diabetes. This means that black women, even when lean, have a higher risk of developing insulin resistance, which leads to excess fat storage in the body if not properly treated. Blacks May Have a "Thrifty Gene" Causing Them to Eat More There is a so-called thrifty gene that helps the body to function on a minimal amount of food. Some researchers believe that African Americans inherited such a gene from their African ancestors. Years ago, this gene enabled Africans, during "feast and famine" cycles, to use food energy more efficiently when food was scarce. People possessing the thrifty gene, which includes African Americans, have a problem in that their built-in appetite suppressant (leptin) doesn't seem to work. Apparently, this gene has lingered from former times when food was not readily available. These people became "leptin resistant," which means their bodies ignore hormonal messages to stop eating and to stop storing fat. This happened because when food was not readily available, their bodies adapted to hold on to fat stores so they could remain alive in those lean times.

Black Women Can Carry More Weight and Still Be Healthy

According to a report by Reuters Health, in a 2011 study conducted by Peter T. Katzmarzyk, associate executive director for population science, and his colleagues at the Pennington Biomedical Research Center, black women can carry more weight than white women and still be considered healthy. Katzmarzyk's group calculated the body mass indexes (BMIs) and measured the waist circumferences of over six thousand men and women of all races to look for the threshold at which weight becomes significantly associated with disease. According to the National Institutes of Health's Clinical Guidelines on the Identification, Evaluation, and Treatment of Overweight and Obesity in Adults, a BMI of 30 or higher is linked to more cases of high cholesterol, diabetes, and high blood pressure. But Katzmarzyk found that the cutoff does not seem to hold true for black women. While there was no racial difference for men, Katzmarzyk showed that for black women, the risk didn't increase until they reached a BMI of 33. Dr. Katzmarzyk thought a possible reason for the contrast might be the difference in the way body fat is distributed in women among the races. So, being skinny (with a low BMI) does not indicate a healthy body, but rather, getting healthy should be the focus of our weight-loss efforts. Getting a healthy body is key to having a beautiful body.

Many Black Women Are Prone to Emotional Eating

Many black women have had to become heads of households, hold down multiple jobs, and raise kids alone. Eating may become a way to deal with the stress and disappointments of life. But unfortunately, weight gain leads to chronic illness. Mortality rates for black women are higher than that for any other racial/ethnic group for nearly every major cause of death, including heart disease, lung cancer, and breast cancer. We are the lifegivers, the caregivers, and think it is our job to take care of everyone but ourselves. However, self-love demands that we take care of ourselves first, so we can give to others from our abundance. We must become accountable to ourselves. Many black women feel that being thick or "phat"—"pretty hot and tempting"—is cute or sexy. However, we must know when phat is actually fat that needs to be burned away to reveal a slim, healthier body. To my sistas, it's time to lose weight and save your life; you've got a lot of living left to do.

Motivation For A New Body And A New You

If you love yourself and have confidence in who you are, you'll begin to send a signal to others that you have value and deserve respect. Loving yourself first sends a clear message that you are to be recognized, celebrated, appreciated, and loved. Sometimes our sense of self-worth or self-esteem is shaped by the people in our inner circle. Some of us have family members and friends ruining our self-esteem every day. Even if they are your flesh and blood, try to remove yourself from their presence as much as possible. Hurtful words negate any progress toward self-worth and self-love.

Let Self-Love Heal Your Mind, Body, and Spirit

Self-love is key to maintaining your healthy, ideal weight. The body has a natural ability to create and maintain the perfect weight for you as long as you are aligned with your true self. For in your true self is everything that is good and perfect about you. By getting back to the truth of who you really are, the real you, you will get to a place where all your problems with weight begin to disappear. Only the power of love can help you find your true self. You have to understand love, a power that is greater than your own. In fact, it's greater than any addiction or eating disorder that you may have. Learning to love will allow you to overcome the power of hate because the truth is that unhealthy eating is an act of self-hate.

The power of love is perfect, healthy, all-knowing, self-healing, and abundant. In contrast, the power of fear is destructive, chaotic, and lacking. It expresses itself as an impostor, causing you to act against your true nature. You have to grow spiritually to understand the power of both love and fear. Both of them are always present and active, but one wishes you health and happiness and the other wishes you death and destruction. Self-love is essential to survival. There is no successful, authentic relationship with others without self-love. We cannot nurture others from a dry well. It is not selfish or self-indulgent. We have to take care of our needs first so we can give to others from our abundance. You will have to love yourself and love your body. Whether you feel fat or overweight, you have to love your body now, unconditionally. If you can't love your body now, then you can't truly love yourself unconditionally. If you can't love your body because you don't like the way it looks, then know that the reasons you became overweight were not all your fault. But now that you have new knowledge about healthy eating, it's time to forgive yourself and others so you can let go of your old body and move toward your slimmer, healthier body.

When you understand the power of love, you can actually love food and make it your friend rather than your enemy. Food nourishes and sustains you; it cements your relationships with family members and friends. Food is meant to be eaten and enjoyed . . . but in moderation. You are not a slave to food. You eat when you are hungry, but you can leave food alone if you are not. The only way to attain a healthy relationship with food is to learn to love it and ensure that the food you put into your body loves you back: it fuels you, nourishes you, and supports your optimal health and vitality. A candy bar does not love you—it's full of sugar and processed chemicals that harm your body. The people who made it don't love you, either—they are just trying to make money by selling you a product. Chemicals and processed foods lead to poor health, sickness, food allergies, ailments, and other diseases, none of which I would classify as "loving" conditions. So, if you are in a place where you still desire candy, that just means that you're still growing spiritually and have not reached your highest, true self. When you do, you won't desire foods that are harmful to your health.

Foods that love you are those that contribute to your health and wellness, such as fruits, nuts and seeds, and vegetables. These healthy, natural foods make your body stronger and able to fight illness and disease and have beauty and vibrancy. Natural, healthy foods make your body strong, fight illness, restore your body, produce beautiful skin, revitalize your mind, give you energy, slow the aging process, and will taste so much better than you can imagine once your taste buds have been reprogrammed. You have to be deliberate about finding healthy foods because unhealthy foods are readily available and easily accessible. But in some instances, I bet you have driven right by the farmers' market or health food store. It's time to make a stop there and begin to change your life.

Don't stress about trying to stop eating unhealthy foods at the beginning of your journey. It is a process that involves breaking your addictions to the many unhealthy foods you eat and think you "love" today. Just be aware of exactly what you're eating and know that there will come a day when you will no longer love foods that don't love you. For me, I overcame my addiction to sugar, sweets, and junk food over time by taking gradual steps. Instead of eating regular chocolate chip cookies with refined white sugar, I began to eat sugar-free cookies that contained artificial sweeteners. Although they were not very healthy, due to either the white flour, trans fats, or artificial sweeteners they contained, they did help me break my addiction to white refined sugar. However, a few months later, once I learned about the dangers of artificial sweeteners and trans fats, I stopped eating sugar-free cookies as well. You will find the right approach for how you transition to more healthy foods that is right for you.

For some people, overeating is a way to cope with painful feelings and emotions. Being overweight and overeating tends to be a relationship issue. You hide behind your weight issues. You have built a wall around yourself, making you unavailable to new friendships and love. To begin loving your body and your true self, post the following affirmative statements on a note card and read them every day before you leave for work:

1. I will have a loving relationship with food. I know that food is a gift from God that I am grateful for because it nourishes my body.

2. I am thankful for my body and look forward to a slimmer, healthier body as I become more enlightened about healthy eating.

3. I will not be afraid to get on the scale because the number that I weigh isn't as important as the overall healthiness of my body. A healthy body is a beautiful body.

4. I will not be ashamed of my body, for it is just the house for my spiritual and mental self; it does not define my true self.

5. I will forgive myself and other people. No more arguing and fighting, only letting go of stresses, failures, and disappointments.

To take your first step toward attaining self-love, you need to evaluate your self-image. Your self-image comes from and is reflected by the thoughts and feelings you have formed and integrated throughout your lifetime. A poor self-image leads to unsuccessful, self-defeating behavior that negatively affects your relationships and overall health. If you lack self-love and treat yourself as unimportant, others will see you as unimportant as well. If you feel yourself unworthy of the time and effort required to lose weight, then it is unlikely that you will grow healthier and happier.

If you are constantly worrying about your weight and always have negative thoughts and feelings that make you unhappy with yourself, it's time to break out of that cycle. If you catch yourself saying negative things to yourself or about yourself, stop and replace those thoughts with positive ones. Say the positive thought out loud. As an example, if you're thinking, "my stomach is so huge," stop yourself and say, "I am excited about how beautiful my body will be when I lose a few pounds." The more you practice this method, the more you begin to change your inner life. Don't allow negative thoughts to linger in your mind. Be diligent about pushing negative thoughts out of your mind and instantly replacing them with thoughts that are encouraging or positive. Don't be wishy-washy about your positive statements, either. Don't say, "I hope to lose weight" or "I'm trying to lose thirty pounds." Instead, say, "I will lose thirty pounds. I will have a slimmer body that makes me feel sexy." You're not planning, wishing, or hoping—you are doing it! Thoughts and feelings have power that can help or hurt you. Changing your thoughts changes your life.

Beware of Emotional Eating

Do you eat when you're sad, hurt, or lonely? Emotional eating almost always leads to inappropriate eating. Without realizing it, you may be caught in a vicious cycle of "living to eat," not "eating to live." Just the same as a drug or alcohol addict, you have to make sure that you don't use food to escape your problems. Food should be seen for what it is: fuel for the body to give it energy and vitality. An important way to address emotional eating is to learn the difference between emotional hunger and physical hunger. This is absolutely key.

Sometimes our relationship with food is an emotional one rather than a physical one. Sometimes we eat to fill an emotional gap or some other negative emotion. But no food, cracker, cake, ice cream, or pie can satisfy emotional hunger. Emotional hunger comes on suddenly—I must eat something now. But you rarely feel satisfied or full, and so you just keep eating and eating until the entire bag of chips or pint of ice cream is gone. If the hunger comes on after an argument or a negative emotion, then it is emotional hunger. You need to learn to deal with the emotions head on. Physical hunger comes about gradually about every three to four hours. Watch the clock. If you ate a meal and were full one hour ago and then feel a sudden need to eat something, it's probably emotional hunger.

Dealing with your emotional issues will help you improve your relationship with food. To deal with your emotions, you must come to understand that the bad things that have happened in your life have probably been floating around in your mind for years, and because you try to suppress these feelings, as most of us do, they have never been properly processed. When we dwell on the sad events of our lives, they get etched in our minds and stuck in our bodies, weighing us down emotionally. We must process these experiences and let them go. If we don't, the negative emotions become toxic to our emotional and physical body. Sad or painful experiences are meant to teach us lessons we needed to learn so that we could grow and mature as a person—they are not meant to linger for years and years. Just as we can get rid of toxic wastes in the body, we can get rid of toxic emotions. Instead of eating to distract ourselves from bad feelings, we need to process and eliminate them—just like the body does with food: it takes the nutrients it needs and expels the rest.

Part of expelling negative emotions involves forgiveness, of yourself and others. Authors Stephen Kendrick and Alex Kendrick discuss forgiveness in their book The Love Dare in the following terms: Forgiveness doesn't clear anyone of blame. It doesn't clear their record with God. It just clears you of having to worry about how to punish them. When you forgive another person, you're not turning them loose, but turning them over to God, who can be counted on to deal with them His way. You're saving yourself the trouble of arguing and fighting. It's not about winning and losing anymore. It's about letting go.

Tips for Staying Motivated

In order to ensure success on the DHEMM System, you may want to follow these tips to stay motivated and committed. Have an attitude of self-forgiveness: You must forgive yourself for the poor and destructive eating habits you've had for so many years. You are like many others in that you have been on the Standard American Diet. However, you cannot move forward in losing weight permanently and restoring optimal health without self-forgiveness. Additionally, you must also forgive friends, family, and others who have fed you an unhealthy diet over the years, as they probably didn't know any better and did the best they could with what they knew at the time. You will sometimes make bad decisions in terms of what you eat. We all lose control and make bad food choices, but it is important to know that one bad decision doesn't have to turn into two or three. The key to weight loss and staying confident is to decrease the number of bad decisions you make on a daily basis.

Make your health a priority: You must begin thinking differently. First, decide that your health is one of the top priorities in your life. Know that your body is naturally thin. If you prepare your mind and absorb the knowledge offered to you in this book, you will have all the power you need to become your best self and transform your life in every way. Even if you are a busy mom or high-powered career executive, know that today begins the journey toward your most amazing, beautiful self. It is time to treat your body as the greatest gift that you have. It is time to shine as the person you were always meant to be. When you have a healthy and positive energy in life, amazing things like love, joy, success, and wealth come your way. Every interaction at work, church, home, or in the streets can be simply magnetic. Get healthy, lose weight, and watch your entire life begin to change for the better.

List ten reasons why you want to lose weight: Give serious thought to this list and ensure that each reason reflects your true goals and desires and that the list is meaningful to you. The reasons should be highly personal and not meant to please anyone but yourself. These become your personal motivators. Read them every day. You may even want to post them at work or carry them in your purse or wallet on an index card. You will need to remind yourself of these motivators to keep yourself focused.

Visualize your goals: What will your life look like when you're thinner and healthier? Visualize your perfect body and get comfortable with the idea it will be yours by the end of this program. Everything in life is made up of energy, including your thoughts. Positive thoughts attract positive energy. Negative thoughts attract negative energy. What you think is what you become. If you think of yourself as slim and healthy, you will begin to move in the direction of being thin and healthy. Don't think about being overweight; think about being thin. See yourself as having an attractive, sexy, energetic body. Allow your thoughts to work with your efforts of changing your eating habits so that you accelerate your progress, having everything in your life working with you, not against you.

Engage in positive self-talk: Thoughts and feelings turn into actions, and actions into reality. Remember, you are beginning a new section in your life. Let me encourage you right now to get started with your journey. Many ask, "How do I start?" or "How do I get there?" Well, it begins with positive self-talk. You want to stop thinking and saying negative things about yourself. You are not fat, lazy, ugly, or sick. Your true self is naturally thin, beautiful, and healthy. If you have negative thoughts about yourself, you'll attract negative people and outcomes in your life. If you say that you can never lose weight, you're exactly right: you won't. If you say you can, your subconscious mind believes that and begins to move your actions in the direction of losing weight.

Don't get obsessed with weighing yourself every day: Don't let your bathroom scale ruin your motivation. Frequent weighing can be confusing, so focus on how your clothes look and feel on your body. Scales are reliable over the long haul but give you inaccurate day-to-day reads. Weight fluctuations can be caused by hormonal changes or fluid shifts and can lead to unnecessary disappointment. It can show gains or losses that are not there because most basic scales can't tell the difference between fat, muscle, and water weight. Your weight also fluctuates by several pounds throughout the day, and weighing yourself too much will only be confusing and discouraging. Plan on weighing yourself only once a week at the same time of day and wearing the same clothing or no clothing (naked is best). Focus on losing inches and on how you begin to feel, not just on pounds. With this program, you will be doing great things for your body and health. The number on the scale will take care of itself. Be happy with losing one to two pounds per week. If you do this for two months, you will be down by sixteen pounds.

Focus on losing body fat, not just weight: It's fine to have a weight goal to use as a guideline, but also focus on measuring and monitoring overall body fat as a percentage of overall weight. This will ensure that you lose fat, not muscle. Healthful body-fat percentages for men begin at about 8 percent, 22 percent for women. These percentages will keep you in a healthy, safe zone that will lower your risk for disease. If you only have a regular scale and want to get detailed body-fat measurements, you can invest in a home body-fat scale. A decent one will cost you about $100 to $200. I own one by Tanita that measures weight, body-fat percentages, and muscle mass and helps me get the best picture of my overall health. Once you begin to measure your body fat, you will be able to track the loss of the thing you really want to lose.

Take a picture: Looking at before and after pictures of your new body can be highly motivating. Of course, you'll be getting comments and compliments from friends, family, and coworkers, but nothing is as special as seeing with your very own eyes your new healthy, beautiful body. Health is important, but I understand your need to improve your physical appearance as well. So get out the camera and take photos as you progress along your weight-loss journey. The reason some people look and feel better than others is that they work at it. Why do you think celebrities look so fabulous despite their age? It's because they are constantly thinking about their appearance. Their livelihood depends upon how good they look. However, anyone can commit to looking fabulous all the time.

You can make the choice to eat whole, healthy foods instead of junk foods, stay active, drink lots of water, and get plenty of rest and relaxation. Yes, it takes more work and discipline to look great as you age, but you will reap the benefits of being your best, beautiful self.

CHAPTER 5

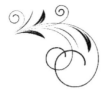

REDUCING DAILY STRESS AND ENHANCING SLEEP QUALITY

S tress is a process that happens when people respond to environmental and psychological stressors that generate challenge or danger. Stress stimulates the "fight or flight" center in the brain, which bring about the release of stress hormones such as catecholamine and cortisol. The catecholamine increase our breathing rate to provide more oxygen to muscles, elevate heart rate and blood pressure, and mobilize fat into the blood for extra energy. Muscles also can become tense, and people under stress often find that their mouths become dry and they begin sweating. In addition, cortisol, another stress hormone, helps store fat and releases sugar into the blood.

The stress response is not always generated by the situation alone—the anticipation of a potential stressor can also have a significant impact on how stress affects an individual. A moderate amount of stress can add interest to daily life and can help us adapt to change, but too much stress has been shown to contribute to a range of health problems, such as heart attack, gastrointestinal problems, hypertension, stroke, diabetes, cancer, tuberculosis, insomnia, pneumonia, influenza, headaches, and an increase in belly fat. There are three main types of stressors: cataclysmic stress, personal stress, and daily stress. A cataclysmic stressor occurs infrequently but is typically life changing. For example, major floods, abnormally cold weather, tornadoes, and plane and train crashes greatly disrupt people's lives and can typically bring about a significant stress response. Personal stressors are usually infrequent but can be equally stressful: the death of a loved one or going through a painful divorce has been shown to generate stress. Daily stressors involve the frustrations that many of us experience, such as commuting in busy traffic, dealing with incompetent coworkers, having too much to do in too little time, and so forth. These stressors can occur frequently throughout the day and have the ability to constantly generate a stress response.

The Effect of Stress on Belly Fat

The major stress hormone that leads to increased deposits of belly fat is cortisol; at high levels in the circulation, this chemical messenger tells the liver to release sugar into the blood, bringing about an increase in blood insulin levels. Constant high levels of cortisol and insulin in the blood encourage fat accumulation and an increase in belly fat.

How to Cope with Stress

There are a number of ways to cope with stress, including taking direct action against and seeking information about the stressor, inhibiting stressful actions, and employing general stress-management habits. For example, if a person's job is his or her main source of stress, then the best solution would be to find another job. Unfortunately, for most people, this is not practical, so they have to find a way of coping with the stress generated by their jobs. If driving in morning traffic is stressful, then a way to cope might be to get information about traffic flow during different times of the day, to provide options for decreasing the stressful effects of traffic.

Another coping mechanism is to stop fighting the stressor and accept it; this is called inhibiting the stressor. It does not get rid of the stressor but saves the energy and effort required for coping with it. For example, rather than getting angry every time you find yourself mired in morning traffic, you could accept that city roads will always be busy during rush hour and play music to help you relax rather than get upset. Finally, if a stressor cannot be removed or inhibited, stress management offers a number of strategies and techniques to reduce or stop the deleterious effects of exposure to daily stressors. Read on and learn how to use stress-management skills such as controlled breathing, muscle relaxation, and imagery to avoid becoming agitated.

Stress Management

Stress management typically involves managing stressors wherever possible, modifying your perception of stressful situations, developing stress-resistance resources, controlling stress reactions, controlled breathing, muscle relaxation, and imagery. More information on these strategies can be found in Minding the Body, Mending the Mind by Joan Borysenko. From a belly fat perspective, the most important strategies include the use of exercise and the development of controlled breathing, muscle relaxation, imagery, and time-management skills to cope with stress.

Controlled Breathing

Controlled breathing is a stress-management technique that concentrates on slowing and optimizing your breathing. Rapid breathing quickly produces a number of unwanted physiological responses, such as an elevated heart rate and feelings of dizziness. A warm, darkened, carpeted room is recommended when learning how to control your breathing and muscle tension. You should lie on your back with your arms by your side; you can lie on the floor or a firm bed. Make sure that your clothing is not tight or uncomfortable. Finally, make sure you do not have any injuries that cause discomfort when lying in this position. Now follow the steps listed below.

1. Close your eyes and focus your thoughts on your breathing.

2. Slow your breathing and take deep, even breaths. Focus all your thoughts on the air as it enters your nasal passage and progresses deep into your lungs. If extraneous thoughts enter your mind, push them aside and refocus all your attention on your breathing.

3. Now concentrate on your breathing cue word: relax. As you say the word in your mind, breathe in on the re and out on the lax. One cycle should take about 5 seconds—2.5 seconds breathing in, and 2.5 seconds breathing out—which equates to twelve breathing cycles per minute. Practice using this cue for three breathing cycles. Remember, slowly breathe in on the re and slowly breathe out on the lax.

4. If thoughts enter your mind or noises come to your attention, push them aside and refocus all your concentration on your breathing.

5. As you practice the muscle relaxation technique in the next section, try to monitor and control your breathing throughout the session using your cue word: relax.

Muscle Relaxation

Muscle relaxation is a technique that systematically releases all the tension in your skeletal muscles. As with the controlled breathing technique, you should lie on your back with your arms by your side in a warm, darkened room. Try to wear comfortable, nonrestrictive clothing. Follow the instructions below to learn how muscle relaxation is performed for the whole body.

1. Lie on your back on a carpeted floor or on a firm bed. Support your head with a small cushion. Allow your legs and arms to stretch out. If you suffer from lower back problems, place a rolled-up blanket under your knees.

2. To begin, complete a body tension check by monitoring all your muscle groups for excessive muscle tension. Close your eyes and scan the muscles in your body from your head to your feet. Try to sense which of your muscles are tense. Don't forget about your breathing; it should be slow and even.

3. Now start muscle relaxation: tense your fist by curling your fingers as tight as you can for fifteen seconds. Hold the tension and focus on it; then release by relaxing your hands and letting your fingers slowly uncurl. Notice the warm, tingling sensation of relaxed muscles, compared with the earlier feeling of tension.

4. Next, focus on your biceps: Create tension in these upper-arm muscles for fifteen seconds by lifting both hands to the shoulders and tightening the biceps. Try to keep your hands relaxed. Now release the tension in your biceps by relaxing them and letting your arms slowly return to your sides.

5. Now tense your neck muscles by contracting and pushing the back of your neck into the pillow for fifteen seconds. Hold the tension, focus on it, and then release it by relaxing your neck.

6. Tense your facial muscles by frowning and gritting your teeth for fifteen seconds. Hold the tension, focus on it, and then release it by relaxing.

7. Now contract your abdominal muscles by tensing and pulling in your stomach for fifteen seconds. Hold the tension, focus on it, and then release it by relaxing.

8. Next, continue with your thighs and buttocks. Tense these muscles tightly for fifteen seconds and then release the tension.

9. Don't forget to focus on your breathing by using your cue word, relax. Take a deep breath on the re, hold your breath, and then release it on the lax.

10. Finish by tensing your lower legs. Keep your eyes closed and contract your feet and lower legs by pushing them into the carpet or bed. Hold the tension for fifteen seconds and then relax. By now you should feel your body getting warm and heavy.

11. Once you have completed the exercise, remain lying down for a while. You may go to sleep, so if you have other things to do, set an alarm clock before you begin.

Imagery Relaxation

Much stress is caused by thinking about negative situations. For some people, relaxing muscles may not be enough, and they must also relax their minds by blocking stressful thoughts and trying to stop worrying. Relaxation imagery involves imagining a relaxing scene by using sight, sound, smell, and touch, which distracts a stressed person from worrying. Choose a relaxing image that you most associate with calmness, peace, tranquility, serenity, and harmony. It might be a real-life scenario, such as walking through the countryside, or a fantasy image, such as drifting along with the clouds. Try to involve all your senses in your imagery, so think about what you can see, hear, touch, and smell. The two practice images described in the instructions below involve clouds and a warm house in winter. Try these images and then develop your own.

When practicing relaxation imagery, a warm, darkened, carpeted room is recommended. You should lie on your back with your arms by your side. Make sure your clothing is not tight or uncomfortable. Also make sure you do not have any injuries that cause you discomfort when lying in this position. Now close your eyes and create the following scene in your mind. You are on a warm, white beach. You are the only person there, the water is calm and green, and the sky is a vivid blue. Focus on the sky. In your mind's eye, you see nothing but blue. Now focus on the green and turquoise colors of the sea. Focus on the smell of the ocean; let the fresh smell of the sea flood your mind. You can feel a gentle sea breeze against your face. Next, focus on the sky, where you can see a small white cloud descending slowly to the beach. The cloud becomes larger until it finally settles under you. You are lying on top of this small cloud. It gently lifts you into the air, and you see the beach becoming smaller and smaller. Your body is becoming lighter and lighter. You feel warm, secure, and relaxed.

Now the cloud descends, and your body is feeling more relaxed. As the cloud touches the beach, you feel warm, heavy, and relaxed. Focus on your breathing. Use your cue word—relax—for two breathing cycles. At the end of the second cycle, open your eyes. You should feel energized and ready for action. Now for your second imagery relaxation exercise: picture a warm house in the middle of winter. With your eyes closed, think about the home: Is it a country house or a town house? Is it modern or old? What sort of houseplants are there? Can you hear the cold wind outside? Can you feel the warmth inside the house? Perhaps you can smell the aroma of your favorite food drifting from the kitchen. Move through each room of the house, concentrating on what you can see, hear, smell, and feel before going on to the next image. Once you have spent a short time exploring, you should know your house so well that you could describe it to someone else.

Note that when you use relaxation imagery techniques, it is not the same as visualizing with your eyes open. When visualizing with your eyes open, you get a sharp, focused picture that remains steady. In contrast, mental images tend to be more fluid—more like ideas of what something looks like rather than a reproduction of reality.

Relaxation On The Go

If stress symptoms seize you in the workplace, following some of the strategies below may help you manage your daily work stressors. At some point during the workday, take a five-minute break when you can:

- sit down and have a healthy snack, such as a piece of fruit;
- remove yourself from your working environment by going outside and walking around;
- find a quiet place and practice the breathing, muscle relaxation, and imagery techniques;
- withdraw to somewhere quiet, close your eyes, and allow your body to rest; or
- if you are working from home, put on a favorite piece of music. Sit or lie down with your eyes closed and listen for a while.

Time Management

Many of the daily hassles that cause us stress on a regular basis are caused by poor time management. Many people are simply not well organized, and trying to do too much in an unplanned fashion can generate the stress response. Characteristics of efficient time management include developing a long-term plan, prioritizing and planning ahead, and using a yearly planner. Planning on a weekly basis involves filling in a weekly planner, using time slots wisely, being flexible, being realistic, and seeking help. Common "time thieves" are procrastinating, wasting time on irrelevant tasks, failing to start a task, drifting off, being a perfectionist, and putting tasks into the too-hard basket. Some easy-to-follow time-management tips include completing small tasks straightaway, breaking tasks into small, manageable units, and developing a goal-setting plan. Goals are really useful for getting things done. Guidelines for effective goal setting include:

- Set specific, measurable goals.
- Set difficult but realistic goals.
- Set short-range goals.
- Set goals based on performance rather than outcomes.
- Set positive goals, not negative ones.
- Identify target dates.

- Record your goals in a yearly planner.
- Evaluate your goals.

An example of short-term goal setting is to complete three weekly twenty minute interval sprinting sessions, eat a piece of fruit each day, and practice muscle relaxation nightly for one week. At the end of the week the completion success of these goals should be evaluated. For example, if practicing muscle relaxation every night was too demanding, then try three times per week. Common obstacles that prevent people from meeting their goals include setting too many goals, making goals too general, setting unrealistic goals, and setting outcome-oriented goals. A goal-setting system allows you to assess your needs, set yourself long-and short-term goals, and evaluate your progress and adjust your goals weekly.

How to Use the Breathing, Muscle Relaxation, Imagery Relaxation, and Time-Management Techniques

You should try all these basic stress-management techniques to see which ones work best for you. Whatever you decide, an effective way of learning and performing the relaxation techniques is to make a tape or a script. Simply read out loud and record the scripts in each of the exercises above on a cassette player or using your phone's Record function, and then practice the skills by playing and listening to the recording. Ideally, you should try relaxing daily or at least three times per week. As you develop these relaxation skills, the protocols may be shortened and transferred to more realistic settings, which is called differential relaxation, though this may take weeks. Progression of differential relaxation could be: relaxing in a chair; relaxing in a car or train; relaxing during stressful situations during the day. Learning to monitor and control anxiety and tension can be achieved through a sound goal-setting system and well-structured stress-management skill sessions.

Exercise And Stress Reduction

The autonomic, cardiac, and vascular changes that occur following participation in regular aerobic exercise are well documented. For example, low resting heart rate—bradycardia—typically occurs with regular aerobic exercise such as running. Resting heart rates of trained runners are often less than 50 beats per minute. Heart rate during an exercise session is also decreased after training. These changes have prompted researchers to speculate that because regular aerobic exercise makes the body more efficient at handling exercise stress, then at the same time it will also produce a more efficient response to psychological stress. There is mixed evidence, however, to suggest that frequent physical activity may decrease the physiological response to stress in healthy individuals. The major finding appears to be that aerobic fitness is associated with slightly better heart-rate recovery from stress.[2]

A decrease in the stress response has been found in those few studies that have examined men and women at cardiovascular risk, such as people whose parents suffered from hypertension or who have hypertension themselves, and we know that the blunted skeletal muscle blood flow and increased blood pressure response to stress commonly found in the overweight and viscerally obese can be normalized with regular exercise. These results have been derived mainly from studies using steady-state aerobic exercise such as cycling, jogging, and swimming, but the effects of other types of exercise, such as interval sprinting, on the stress response are poorly explored. We have shown that one session of interval sprinting, compared with one of steady-state exercise, produced a significantly greater impact on the autonomic nervous system, as assessed by heart rate and blood levels of catecholamine levels. Regular interval sprinting training also resulted in a significant change in resting cardiovascular and autonomic function.

Given that interval sprinting induces a significant acute cardiovascular response, it is possible that interval sprinting training may also produce greater adaptations to the stress response. Recently, we examined the effect of interval sprinting on the stress response. We found that twelve weeks of sprinting produced significant differences in cardiovascular and autonomic response during exposure to a laboratory stressor. Specifically, men who performed twelve weeks of interval sprinting experienced a significant reduction in heart rate during a challenging computer task. Exercisers, compared with a group of volunteers, also showed decreased stiffness of their large arteries and increased muscle blood flow during stress. There are a number of other ways to use exercise to help relieve the stress in our lives. As mentioned earlier, regular involvement in physical activity such as interval sprinting causes the body to adapt to both exercise and psychological stress. We know that exercisers have significantly less incidence of cardiovascular disease and stroke, but how much of this effect is due to a reduced stress response is unknown. Another way of using exercise to buffer the stress response is to use it as a "time-out": after a busy morning at work, taking a fifty-minute jog around a pleasant park at lunchtime may simply distract an individual from the stress of work.

Similarly, participating in twenty minutes of interval sprinting while listening to invigorating music may also direct people's thoughts away from daily stressors. However, more research on the stress-reducing capacity of interval sprinting is needed.

Sleep It Off

Most human behaviors have an obvious purpose. For example, we eat to provide energy for the body and drink water to supply fluid in and around the cells. Up to 30 percent of a person's life may be spent in sleep; however, the physiological function of sleep is unknown. The two main hypotheses to explain why we have to sleep are restoration and protection. The restoration hypothesis suggests that we sleep to restore the energy depletion that occurred during the previous day. However, approximately the same amount of energy is expended while sitting and sleeping.

Moreover, bedridden people sleep more than healthy people. The protective hypothesis suggests that our nervous system carries hardwired behavioral patterns; because we lack adequate night sensors, it is safer to sleep at night.

Whatever the reason for sleeping, it is known that lack of sleep or poor-quality, nonrefreshing sleep has an adverse effect on health; after the common cold, sleep problems are the second-biggest health complaint, and there are over fifty identified sleep disorders. People experiencing regular sleep disruption typically possess greater body and belly fat than people who sleep well. Sleep-deprived people also face greater difficulty losing fat after a diet or exercise intervention. Differences in the number of hours of sleep also influence body composition, as it has been shown that people who sleep less tend to be overweight. Disrupted sleep may change the balance between satiety hormones that control hunger, as sleeping five hours per night results in greater ghrelin and less leptin levels compared with sleeping eight hours.

Leptin, a hormone secreted by fat cells, tells the brain that we have had enough to eat, while ghrelin, secreted from the lining of the gut, transmits the message "I'm hungry!" Thus, sleep deprivation affects body fat accumulation because it makes us hungrier. Increased resting cortisol levels have also been found in people who experience lack of sleep. As a result, sleeping well is very important for helping the body spend longer in fat burning mode than in fat-storing mode.

Mindfulness Meditation

Through mindfulness meditation, we can become more aware of our thoughts. The objective in meditation is to take a step outside of our thoughts and, as an observer, become aware of them. From this perspective, we can pay precise, nonjudgmental attention to the details of our experiences. Mindfulness meditation alleviates stress by helping us practice being present. It also involves reminding us of pleasant experiences from our past, when we have been able to overcome struggle and achieve personal success. There are many forms of meditation, but all have the same general goals. (Tai chi and yoga are forms of moving meditation with long traditions.)

We don't want to get rid of our thoughts, only become aware of them. We aren't trying to change ourselves, but instead become aware of ourselves as we presently are and objectively observe our thoughts, good or bad. Meditation can help us work through the thoughts, enabling us to cope with stress much more effectively. Mindfulness meditation can be particularly helpful in working through our feelings of hunger and cravings for foods. Meditation often only takes twenty to thirty minutes and can be done any time. Cultivate the habit of waking up in the morning, having a class of cold water and beginning your meditation. Three basic aspects are involved in mindfulness meditation: body, breath and thoughts.

Body

First, you want to connect with your body. Find a quiet location where you will not be disturbed for the next twenty minutes. Sit down either on the ground, on a cushion or in a chair. Cross your legs if you are sitting on the ground or on a cushion. If you are sitting on a chair, make sure your feet are placed comfortably on the ground, or on a pillow if your feet do not touch the ground below. It is important that you feel comfortable and relaxed in the position you chose. Rest your hands on your thighs, palms facing down. Gaze down at the floor about six feet ahead of you and focus on the tip of your nose, and then gently close your eyes. Feel your chest becoming open and your back becoming strong.

Begin your meditation sitting in this position. For a couple of minutes, focus on how your body and your environment feel. If your thoughts wander away from your body, gently bring them back to your body and environment. Do this throughout your meditation every time your mind wanders away.

Breath

Once you have begun to relax, start to focus in gently on your breath. Breathe in through your nose to the count of six and exhale through your mouth slowly to the count of six. Pay attention to how your breath feels entering and exiting your body.

Thoughts

As you sit, you may become bombarded by thoughts. Pay attention to these thoughts. If they cause you to experience any negative emotions, try to think back to a time where you experienced similar challenges and remember how it felt to overcome those challenges. Work though these thoughts until your body begins to feel lighter. If you notice that you have become so caught up in your thoughts that you have forgotten where you are, gently bring your thoughts back to your breath.

Sleep hygiene

There are several keys to good sleep hygiene, and none of these involve the use of medication. (Medications disturb the normal sleep architecture, the pattern of REM and non-REM sleep.) Simple but effective ways to improve sleep include the following:

- Sleep in complete darkness.
- Sleep in loose fitting clothes.
- Keep regular sleeping hours.
- Try to get seven to nine hours of sleep each night.
- See the light first thing in the morning.
- Keep your bedroom slightly cool.
- Do not keep a TV in your bedroom.

Move It To Lose It

Getting in touch with your body is especially important when you are trying to lose weight. Emotional eating must be distinguished from true hunger, and boredom from starvation. Subtle alterations in body composition develop and must be recognized. Even how you think about food can change. Being physically active enhances your ability to detect each of these changes.

We were born to move, to be active, and to challenge our bodies. For this reason it is necessary to incorporate into our daily lives activities that elevate heart rate, stretch our muscles, and produce all the beneficial hormonal changes that make losing weight much easier. All of these things are great for the brain and the body, and they just plain feel good once you get used to them! It is no surprise that being active on a regular basis is part of a healthy lifestyle. And to reap the benefits you don't have to be Michael Phelps. Setting aside the time and sticking to it are what really count. Remember the Nike slogan: "Just Do It"? After each session you will feel more energized than you did after the prior one. Although most of us can begin moving in a safe fashion, it is best to get a doctor's okay before starting any exercise program.

A Big Waste of Time?

To properly evaluate the benefits of the Feed Your Brain Lose Your Belly diet and activity program, we tested it in a group of volunteers. When they began the activity part of the program, several of them thought it was going to take a lot of time—time they didn't have to spare. Yet, by the end of the study, those who most ardently resisted the activity program became its staunchest supporters. If you haven't done anything in a while to break a sweat, it can be surprising how winded you become just from walking up a flight of stairs. That's why it makes sense to start slowly, pace yourself, and be comfortable. Otherwise, you might get hurt. When this happens, any activity or exercise program comes to a screeching halt. So, it is better to be the tortoise rather than the hare in this situation, which also helps to ensure that you understand and feel good about your increased level of physical activity. Stressing this approach during the weekly meetings with our volunteers helped remove any anxiety about exercising.

Another recommendation we heard repeatedly was that to facilitate compliance, simplicity and convenience were of paramount importance. Still another suggestion was to choose a friend with whom to exercise (literally an "exercise buddy" to help keep you on the program), to compare notes and to just plain enjoy the experience. This will help keep you on track no matter what the weather is like. The mere sight of a pedometer on one of the study volunteers generated support from coworkers, friends, and relatives, which made it easier to stick with the program. It also created new friends and walking partners. These were welcome and unexpected perks of wearing that funny little box around wherever they went. It was like a "yellow badge of courage." When approached in this manner, working out soon becomes something to look forward to. Believe it or not, you might even start to feel cheated if you miss a few sessions. It can even help with sleep difficulties—both falling asleep and being able to sleep through the night. You'll feel rejuvenated after you get your blood pumping. And stairs will gradually become less of a challenge.

It was for all these reasons that almost everyone felt that including some physical activity in their daily schedule was vital. It also became a personal challenge, with all of the participants pushing themselves to surpass what they had accomplished the prior week. This was easy to measure because all were given pedometers to wear and graphed the number of steps they took every day. A few of our experts were startled to learn how far one can walk without going outdoors—even though getting fresh air was so stimulating. Many of the volunteers for the weight loss study were very heavy and very out of shape. For them, the act of walking to the mailbox was difficult. For these reasons, and because we wished to avoid any injuries, the "program" they followed was quite different than what would be recommended for someone only fifteen or twenty pounds overweight. It was designed to get them moving comfortably and safely, to take the first steps to a healthier life. They know that was the plan, and joining the gym was the next step in the progression. The exercise part of the Feed Your Brain Lose Your Belly diet and activity program includes three types of activity: walking, weight training, and balance and coordination. Walking should be performed three times a week—usually on Monday, Wednesday, and Friday—for 30 to 50 minutes. We recommended that study volunteers perform resistance training twice a week—usually on Tuesday and Thursday—for 20 to 30 minutes. They rotated exercising the three body areas sequentially as follows: (1) upper body strengthening, (2) trunk activity, and (3) lower body strengthening. We were not attempting to make people muscle bound; the goal was to include some "power" training (weight training) that augmented the aerobic benefits of walking.

Weight training is also great for bone health. Approximately ten minutes of balance and agility activities were scheduled whenever time allowed, typically several times per week. Just like they recorded all that they ate, volunteers documented every workout by detailing in a personal logbook what activity had been undertaken. This practice allowed each subject to track his or her progress. The study subjects were counseled to adhere to the activity program but to stay within their comfort zone. This approach was recommended for three reasons: to avoid injuries, to make it easier to stick with the program, and to keep it fun. We suggested levels of activity that were "mild" to "moderate" because we wanted everyone to feel safe and to have a stable foundation from which to build. We were hoping they would achieve a sense of well-being, an improvement in cardiovascular fitness, and enhanced strength and balance—all without stimulating appetite excessively.

Keep It Simple—Walk

Walking was the preferred form of aerobic activity in the clinical study, and it doesn't require a pool, track, or treadmill. Plus, it starts as soon as you step out the front door, so no gym pass is necessary. The local shopping mall was also a favorite venue because it was enclosed, which assured protection from the elements. It provided a safe and well-lit place to walk while also being a great place for people watching. Since we attempted to make our activity program as user-friendly as possible, this was a perfect solution because it allowed everyone to participate and enjoy it. What seemed to work best was walking three times a week on alternating days for 30 to 50 minutes. Each session included a tenminute warm-up and a similar ten-minute cool-down period at the end. Almost everyone started at 30 minutes and slowly extended their time to 45 or 50 minutes. Please note that if you have other health problems or haven't exercised in a while, you may need to start more slowly. If so, don't be discouraged; you'll be surprised at how quickly you will be able to increase your exercise time as your body becomes accustomed to the exertion and as you start to lose weight.

The warm-up and cool-down periods consisted of slower intervals designed to get the blood pumping and make sure there were no injuries. The main exercise segment consisted of a period lasting 10 to 30 minutes depending on where people were in the program. During this segment, the volunteers used one of three approaches. (1) Each time they walked they increased their speed slightly compared to what it had been during the prior session but never to exceed the threshold that made it uncomfortable to carry on a conversation with a walking partner. (2) Others used a different approach consisting of intervals of faster walking (for two to five minutes) alternating with slower intervals. (3) Another method employed (during an individual session) was walking at a slowly increasing rate in a crescendo fashion to a peak speed, followed by a decrescendo back down to the rate at which the person had started.

All of these approaches are fine. Using one method and then another is also acceptable. It is important to mix up any workout regimen to keep it lively. What we stressed was getting into the habit of being active through walking—preferably with a friend—and making it a part of the weekly routine. All study participants wore their pedometers and kept track of the number of steps they took during their walks. These were subsequently entered into their logbooks.

Keep It Simple—Train with Weights

The second component of the activity program involved light resistance training. Working out with weights was usually performed every Tuesday and Thursday around the home, which made it simple for everyone. Easily held household objects weighing up to 20 pounds were identified. They became the "weights" that were hoisted several times a week. Bags of coffee, cans of soup or soda, five-pound bags of flour, sacks of wild birdseed, and plastic one-gallon water containers were easy to locate. Gallon containers are particularly useful because the amount of liquid in them can easily be increased as muscle strength improves. What they weighed could easily be determined by putting them on a bathroom scale. Some items were held in one hand while others required a double-handed grip. Light weights were used initially.

As people became stronger, they progressed to somewhat heavier weights. No weights were necessary for some of the other musclebuilding exercises. Upper body, trunk, and lower body workouts were alternated throughout the week. Weight training is an intense form of exercise. If you have never done anything like it, you might consider seeking help from a certified trainer or an experienced friend. As you become stronger, you will need to use slightly heavier weights. At this point in your reading, it will be helpful to take a moment to go over some terminology that you might not be familiar with. Imagine that you are holding a can of soup in your right hand. A repetition (commonly called simply a rep) is the act of moving the can through a full range of motion of any particular joint, for example, the elbow. A group of repetitions performed sequentially, usually six to ten, is called a set. Usually two sets of any specified exercise were performed for each of three muscle groups. This simple approach takes about twenty minutes to complete.

Let's walk through a typical session.

- Arm and Shoulder Exercises

Arm and shoulder exercises strengthen the biceps muscle, the deltoid muscle, and the triceps muscle.

- The Biceps Muscle

The biceps is the muscle that bends the elbow joint in an upward manner. Its range of motion begins with the arm hanging in a resting position nearly straight down. A can of soup or something slightly heavier is held in the hand. Start bending the elbow up until your hand is near your ear. The motion ends here before being reversed—which means slowly lowering your arm until the elbow is almost straight again. Repeat this six to ten times; that is, complete a set of reps. The other arm is then put through the same group of movements. Perform two sets for each arm. This completes the workout for the biceps muscles.

- The Deltoid Muscle

The deltoid is the muscle that moves the shoulder. When you place your hand on the shoulder, you are feeling the deltoid muscle. With your hand at your side using the same can you just used (keeping the arm straight), slowly raise the hand through an arc out to the side until it is parallel to the ground. You will have moved your hand through a 90- degree arc. Now slowly reverse this motion. That completes one rep. Repeat this movement six to ten times and stop. Perform the same exercises on the other arm. This completes one set. After you perform the second set you will have exercised two muscles.

- The Triceps Muscle

The third muscle is the triceps muscle. It straightens (or extends) the elbow joint. For this exercise, you will need a heavier can, such as a large juice can. Grasp it in both hands and hold it over your head with your arms straight up. Now bend both elbows 90 degrees by lowering the can behind your head. Pause, then straighten your arms again over your head. This is one rep. Repeat six to ten times to complete one set of triceps exercises. After you are rested, repeat the set. This ends the upper body strength training session. It will take about twenty minutes to complete.

- Leg Exercises

Leg exercises strengthen the calf muscle, the quadriceps muscle (also known as the "quad" or the thigh muscle), and the hamstring muscle.

- The Calf Muscle

Grasp a plastic one-gallon water container in each hand. Start with them only half filled. In a comfortable standing position, start by rocking up onto your toes. Hold that for two seconds, then roll back down onto the soles of your feet. This constitutes one rep. Repeat six to ten times. Wait a minute or two, then do a second set.

- The Quad Muscle

Lunges are a good way to build up strength in the quadriceps muscle. I would suggest not holding any weights the first several times you perform this exercise.

Try to perform a series of lunges, first on the left side then the right. Start in a comfortable standing position with your feet side by side. While keeping your back upright, take one step forward. As you do, lower your pelvis until your front knee is bent almost 90 degrees. Hold this position for up to three seconds. Straighten up, take the next step, and repeat the maneuver on the other leg. Repeat six times. This constitutes one set. If you feel confident proceeding, try another set.

After you become comfortable with lunges performed in this manner, you are ready to try and carry hand weights. To get started, try using light weights in each hand something the size of a can of soup might be best. Perform the lunges as you did previously, this time using the hand weights.

- The Hamstring Muscle

Knee-flexion training exercises the hamstring muscles. A simple way to strengthen them is by sitting on the edge of a chair. Sit up straight with your feet on the ground and your heels touching the chair. Starting with one foot, press and hold your heel firmly against the front of the chair. Hold this position for four or five seconds, then relax. Repeat six to ten times with the same foot. Now perform the same series using the other foot. If you can comfortably repeat another set, do so. This completes the lower extremity strength training.

- Trunk Exercises

Trunk training typically strengthens your side muscles, abdominal muscles, and back muscles. Start in a comfortable standing position with your feet about a foot apart, then place your hands out to your side. This is the neutral position for the three trunk exercises below. Start without using any weights. The weight of your body will act as the resistance. When you are ready, try holding light weights (two-to five-pounds) in each hand.

- The Side Muscles

For the sides, slowly lower one shoulder laterally to about a 45-degree angle. Hold it for three seconds, then perform the same maneuver in the opposite direction. This constitutes one rep. Perform six to ten reps. Repeat the set.

- The Abdominal Muscles

For the abdominal muscles, start upright in the neutral position. Then lean backward 20 to 30 degrees until you can feel your abdominal muscles tighten. Hold that position for three seconds then return to neutral. That is one rep. As above, repeat six to ten times. This is one set. After a brief rest, repeat the set. This completes the abdominal exercises.

- The Back Muscles

Starting from the same neutral standing position described above, bend forward about 45 degrees. You will feel the muscles in your back tighten. Hold this position for three seconds, then slowly straighten up. This constitutes one rep. Perform six to ten reps. After a brief rest, repeat the set. It is important to do all of the resistance exercises slowly to gain full advantage of the challenge presented by each motion. Doing them rapidly creates momentum that reduces the difficulty of each exercise. If it is too difficult to do an exercise slowly, lighten the weight until you become stronger and can increase it again. When you have become comfortable with these exercises, you can begin to include others. There are many websites and other exercise guides you can use to become more adept at weight training. I also suggest joining a gym and working with a qualified trainer.

Keep It Simple—Improve Balance and Coordination

The third component of the exercise program incorporates activities that improve balance and coordination. Examples include walking on irregular paths, jumping rope, playing ping-pong, and hopping first on one foot, then the other. Although these activities don't sound very difficult, all of our volunteers felt they were important. I believe they also help prevent injuries by improving balance skills. They can be practiced separately or performed while walking.

Positive Feedback

This approach to exercise and activity was enthusiastically supported by everyone. It made them all feel better both mentally and physically, helped them burn calories, and created an esprit de corps among the group. The recommendations were the same for each participant. However, they were personalized and adapted to accommodate various schedules and routines. Each of the volunteers felt that this was a fun and useful part of the program and enthusiastically suggested that you incorporate a similar version in your activity regimen. Much to their surprise, by the conclusion of the clinical trial, many of the participants had progressed sufficiently to take the next step and join a gym or recreation center for exposure to a greater variety of aerobic and resistance machines. An unexpected benefit of the "move it to lose it" program was the increased zest for life that was engendered. Hopefully you'll experience that as well.

Dealing With The Mind-Body Challenges Of Losing Weight

Ten years ago, one in four Americans was obese. Now that number is one in three! On average, being obese usually means being about twenty-five pounds beyond just being overweight. Suppose you are a middle-aged female who is about 5'5" and your ideal weight is 125 pounds. If you weigh 150 pounds, you meet the criteria for being overweight. If you weigh 175 pounds, you are considered obese. About one-third (or more) of the weight of people who fall into this category is fat tissue.

This means they are carrying around almost sixty pounds of fat— upstairs, downstairs, while working, and even when exercising. No wonder it takes a toll on their bodies and joints. Imagine carrying a sixty-pound pack everywhere you go! If you were short of breath, it wouldn't be surprising. But that is exactly what many of us are doing. About 200 million Americans are overweight, and half of them (100 million) are obese. Carrying excess weight is also associated with an array of serious health issues, including diabetes, high blood pressure, stroke, heart attack, heart failure, certain types of cancer, gallstones, gout, osteoarthritis, and sleep apnea. As if those aren't frightening enough, we can now add memory loss and Alzheimer's disease to this daunting list. Needless to say, accumulation of body fat is a huge and growing problem.

In addition to taking a toll on us personally, the fiscal burden it imposes on the country's health-care budget is staggering. Annual health costs attributed to being overweight currently exceed $100 billion. This represents almost 10 percent of the total medical spending in this country. There are even current predictions suggesting that most Americans will be overweight within the next ten years! With figures (and figures) like these, one might think there is something in the drinking water. Perhaps that is true. But there is definitely something in the food we eat. While genes clearly may predispose certain individuals to excessive energy storage (meaning fat storage), the emergence of widespread obesity has only recently become a problem. Surprisingly, not too long ago starvation was a much more pressing concern than obesity.

The Personal Toll of Being Overweight

Gaining significant weight usually takes a long time. It often requires months to reverse the process, if successful, and it isn't nearly as much fun. Large children get teased mercilessly. Adults fare no better. They feel the impact socially, professionally, and medically. It requires tremendous courage to embark on a weight-loss program. At this time, your friends, who should be your biggest advocates, often turn against you. (When you undertake a weight-loss program, it involves facing the fact that you are overweight. Many overweight people can't stand admitting it. When they see their overweight friend start exercising, this realization is sometimes more than they can bear. They react by avoiding the person altogether.) Pursuing such a challenging course can be demoralizing, and going it alone can often prove overwhelming. To make matters worse, losing weight is usually not the only hardship that must be confronted. No one attempting such an arduous quest can be successful without addressing an array of emotional and psychological specters. Deb K, a confirmed yo-yo dieter, will attest to that wholeheartedly.

She first realized she was too heavy when she was a teenager. It was at about the same time that her complexion flared up. At first she was unsure whether the problem was due to stress, boys, or weight gain—or maybe a combination of all three. But weight was clearly a factor. She later became aware of the social impact of being heavy when she was ridiculed by her classmates and had trouble getting dates. As she gained more weight, she soon realized that finding clothes that fit and looked attractive was difficult, so she started wearing looser tops that hung out over her pants in a futile attempt to hide her excess pounds. Later in life she began to have shortness of breath when she walked up more than one flight of stairs. She questioned her doctor about this. He explained that it was because she was carrying around fifty extra pounds and asked her to imagine how she would feel if she had to tote the equivalent of two heavy shopping bags wherever she went. That's when it dawned on her that being overweight could have potentially serious health ramifications. She was well aware that her dad, who had been quite heavy for a long time, had died of a heart attack. The other thing that really bothered her was that she found it impossible to do many things that she had been able to do previously, such as playing tennis and skiing. Her body was failing her!

In addition to the adverse health implications associated with being overweight, how you feel physically can have psychological overtones. Todd D and Marie L said the thing that bothered them the most was the way they felt in their clothes—like stuffed sausages. Several others hated the way their bodies seemed to jiggle when they walked—a perception they were painfully aware of. Each movement was an ominous indicator of these changes—an indicator that was apparent for everyone to see. Occasionally, psychological stressors provide the perfect backdrop for gaining weight. Life is hard enough. Financial worries, caring for aging parents or difficult children, and a myriad of other challenges only make it more difficult. Such was the case for Katrina R, who grew up in an abusive family. It seemed like whatever she did was not quite good enough: her grades were inadequate, her sports performances were not up to par, her bed was never made right, and her closets were too messy. In other words, nothing she did was ever up to expectations. She doesn't remember ever receiving a compliment from her parents, and she subsequently (probably subconsciously) married a man who shared many of her father's traits.

For her, food was more a nutrient for the soul than for the body. It was a reward for what she achieved at work, a comfort for times when she didn't succeed, and punishment for not meeting her own goals. For as long as she could recall, she had considered herself to be an "emotional eater." She received gratification from food, because it was the only positive factor in her life. Unfortunately for her, it contributed to her yearly ten-to fifteen-pound weight gain—adding an unwieldy sixty-one pounds to her petite frame over five years. When she started the clinical trial and had to forego her comfort foods, she was worried about how she would cope without the safety net they provided. Possibly the most poignant reminder of the impact of gaining weight is the realization of the associated health issues and the attendant fragility of life. The potential consequences of these insights made each and every volunteer in the study reflect upon the fact that they might not be there to take care of their aging parents or growing children. This single observation was the most prescient and motivating factor that kept them on the program. Grappling with one's mortality can be intimidating.

How you feel inside your body, the way you relate to people, and how you think about food are all issues that must be dealt with. So you will need to dig deep and be mentally and physically tough. You'll learn a lot about yourself as you proceed with the Feed Your Brain Lose Your Belly diet and activity program. One of the most important tasks you will confront is how you'll react to a new way of eating and a new way of living. Getting in touch with your body will be the first step that will need to be taken during the transformation—and a transformation it will be, because you'll be a different person at the end of the journey.

Get in Touch with Your Body

This phrase means different things to different people, but it is probably the most significant principle that those who stay thin have mastered. When you begin a new way of eating, what is most important is becoming aware of the vague, often unfamiliar signals your body will be generating; understanding what they are telling you; and knowing how to respond appropriately. If you want to be successful at losing weight, getting in touch with your body is essential! A different activity profile, novel dietary recommendations, and alternative nutritional guidelines will combine to produce quite substantial metabolic alterations. Some may occur immediately, whereas others will become apparent only after several weeks. Your body may require some time to adapt to them. It is important to take a moment to understand what these are and how they can influence the way you feel and react. Heightened awareness will facilitate the entire process.

Knowing what to look for makes it easier to discern subtle changes at an earlier stage and to avoid misinterpreting them. To get started let's talk about several of the pathways that will be affected. For any weight-loss program to be successful, you must burn more fat than you store. When you gain weight, you are doing just the opposite—storing more fat than you are burning. To reverse this process, you must change the way your body works. As a result, novel signals will be produced that you may not have experienced previously. You must be aware of them and be able to determine what message they are sending.

Preventing the development of sticky fat cells is an example of one of these changes. Not misunderstanding the new signals your body will be generating is another. This is worth discussing in more detail, because it can derail any diet in a heartbeat. I think it is safe to say that no one is going to stick to a diet if they feel hungry all the time. However, there are certain signals your body will be producing that might be misconstrued as hunger if you're not aware of them. As was mentioned previously, a falling blood sugar level can generate a hunger response if the fall is far enough. As the sugar level decreases, the body will tap into its fat stores. If it is unable to access its internal energy stores, it will need to tap into its external energy supply, which means eating more. This response is due to the hunger signal that is generated by the brain. If you are following the guidelines of the Feed Your Brain Lose Your Belly diet, as your sugar level falls, your fat cells will release fat for the body to burn. It will take over for glucose as a fuel source, there won't be an energy shortage, and you won't need to eat at that time. However, whether you end up needing to eat or you tap into your fat cells and don't get hungry, both scenarios begin with a falling blood sugar level. This blood sugar change makes the brain aware of the potential need for some form of nutrition in the future. For this reason, as you make the transition from sugar to fat burning, your body will sense the change, and you will become aware of it. However, it should not be interpreted as hunger, but merely as how the transition to the fat-burning state feels. It is a perception that should be viewed positively because it is how weight is lost, and it is a transition we should be making multiple times each day. If you are not aware of how it feels, it might easily be misconstrued as true hunger and will prompt an eating response. That is the last thing you want to do if losing weight is your goal. So, be cognizant of what to look for and don't end up thinking the transition to the fat-burning state is a hunger signal.

As you have seen, to lose weight without being hungry requires successfully making the transition from using external calories (meaning the food we eat) to internal calories (the fat stored in our pantries). Once this occurs, we're home free, because many of us have enough fat to last for a very long time. The most efficient ways to facilitate this transition are to choose foods that contain slow-release carb sources and to add brain-healthy fats to each meal. The slow-release carbs blunt the fall in sugar while the brain healthy fats speed up fat burning. They work together to make the conversion from burning glucose to burning fat much easier. The transitions from one fuel to another are small and appetite is suppressed. However, a subtle transition still occurs. For this reason, it is important to remember that such a diet can produce feelings that may be misinterpreted as early signs of hunger. However, they are not signs of starvation or lack of food, but merely reflect a transition in the fuel mixture from carbohydrate to fat.

This is why being in touch with your body and knowing how to interpret what you feel is critical—it helps differentiate a normal metabolic transition from other perceptions. Probably the most meaningful way to describe this subtle distinction is to characterize it like the difference between wanting to eat and needing to eat. With this perspective, it is possible to identify the physiological shift from the fat storing to the fat-burning state—the condition associated with weight loss! Nicole R summed it up nicely when she said, "I never felt hungry, because there was no need to be hungry!"

Now for the Hard Part—Dealing with the Emotions

Learning how your body is going to react when you start making better food choices and begin an exercise program allows you to be ideally poised to tackle all the emotional challenges you will be facing. The volunteers in our clinical study went through similar adversities and have provided compassionate perspectives that they found helpful. If you look around, the first thing that should strike you is that you are not alone! No matter how out of shape, overweight, or depressed you are about being too heavy, there are many others who are in worse shape and need to lose weight even more urgently than you do. You should also acknowledge that losing weight might not be easy for you. However, I suggest you keep in mind the fact that many people have walked in your shoes, and a number of them have achieved their goals!

While success is a great motivator, there will be times when, regardless of what you do, you find yourself stuck on a dreaded weight-loss plateau. This produces many negative reactions including desperation, anxiety, depression, and fear of failure. To maintain your sanity at times like these it helps to accept the fact that you will be dealing with a multitude of raw emotions. Sometimes that is the most difficult thing to realize.

Self-Esteem Is Key—Don't Let Your Weight Define You as a Person!

A number of the study volunteers had issues regarding self-esteem. As a result, many of them shared the misguided belief that "I am not thin enough = I am not good enough." Ostensibly this makes no sense, yet it is ingrained in our culture. Consider how models, actresses, and other females in various ads are depicted. Whether they are advertising cars, cosmetics, beer, or cell phones, it seems that thinner is better. Because we live in an age when this type of information dominates TV, movies, magazines, and the Internet, we are all exposed both consciously and subconsciously to the association of a waif-like body with success, beauty, and power.

With this type of upbringing and subliminal messaging, it is not surprising that young girls (and boys as well) develop problems of selfesteem as they mature. As time goes by, additional life stressors such as finances, work, health, and family-related issues may conspire to cause one's body image to become increasingly difficult to contend with. Maddie W was so troubled by how she reacted to her weight gain that she was prescribed an antidepressant. Incidentally, among their many other side effects, antidepressants can be associated with weight gain and, like all medications, should only be taken under a doctor's care. In Maddie's situation, her medication made it more difficult for her to lose weight. This contributed to losing her sense of self-worth and the downward spiral that ensued. Once this type of thing happens, reversing the process can be extremely difficult.

The good news for Maddie was that she had a great sense of humor and even did some stand-up comedy. That provided her with a sounding board for her emotions and allowed her to vent about her life, her circumstances, and how they made her feel. Luckily, at one of her shows she met a wonderfully supportive young man who convinced her that she was indeed a good person. This sincere gesture of support and honesty allowed her to start feeling much better about herself and what she could contribute to society. Once she realized that there was so much more to life than having a stick figure, she started feeling better about herself and became much more successful at meeting her weight loss goals.

How it feels to be overweight is never good, but it seems to affect us all quite differently and produces various responses. It might even generate different feelings at different times in one's life, depending on the situation and history of past experiences. Trudy K referred to her weight gain as an indication of inadequacy. She said if she was unable to control what she put in her mouth, there was not much hope of successfully controlling anything else. It was as if gaining weight was a metaphor for many of the failures she had suffered over the years—a different manifestation of the same underlying pathology.

Determine What Is Important in Your Life

Concerns about her weight had plagued June D for a long time. Her friends were "on her case," and she was in a tizzy about what to do. She was finding it increasingly difficult to walk the eighteen holes of golf she played every Saturday without feeling somewhat winded. Bending over to do the yard work she loved so dearly was now a chore as well. Her knees had begun popping and had started aching over the past six months. Though she was only fifty years old, it seemed to her that her body was starting to give out. Working in a bank where she spent most of the time at a desk didn't help the situation. Being a "professional" woman was all she ever wanted. And she was good at what she did. Whenever a problem arose, she was the "go-to girl" for a creative solution. Worried that she was even losing that talent, she started feeling overwhelmed. It seemed like a number of factors had coalesced to make her feel inept, inadequate, and intimidated. This was uncharted territory. People had always looked up to her and respected her opinion. She felt like she was losing control. About that time she went to visit her daughter Randi, who sensed something was awry. After several attempts, June finally opened up and the two spoke frankly for a few hours. Randi was able to react in an objective manner to her mom's predicament. Following her sage advice, June decided to devote more attention to her own needs. She carved out periods during the week that were designated as "private time"—a particularly important practice that might apply to you, too, because so many people are busy giving to others that they don't take the necessary time to address their own needs. She even resumed her favorite childhood hobby of playing the piano, which helped to rejuvenate her.

And she created some much needed distance between her private life and her professional life. This combined approach also made it much easier for June to focus on her weight-loss program, which was made more enjoyable and successful via a group effort with several of her friends who also wanted to lose weight.

Work at It, Don't Get Depressed, and Accept Help from Others

For a number of reasons, becoming a Big Loser is not an easy accomplishment. You must realize there are numerous ways to get to the finish line, many of which are not direct, predictable, or easy. Just when things are looking good, you might let up and even gain one or two pounds. This has happened to each of our experts, often more than once! Instead of fearing it, it is best to assume it will happen and learn to deal with it. Part of successfully confronting a wrinkle in your plans is having the mental toughness to work through it. This is where your focus should be. The consensus of the group was that if you approach things this way, you won't get depressed or feel overwhelmed. Midway through the weight-loss study Natalie G gained a few pounds. At about that time her young daughter thought she had become pregnant. Working through this situation was almost too much for Natalie to bear. The stress was a real killer, and could have been a diet-breaker as well. Luckily for Natalie, it wasn't.

Marti B made these observations about stress and hunger. "Another thing that was very important to me was distinguishing between how it feels to be hungry and the false sense of hunger that can arise out of stress—a response that doesn't merit eating. That might be the most important thing I learned during the support group meetings. My friends were there to help me. Knowing I was not alone gave me the courage to continue." This shows the dramatic impact a good support system can provide. You're almost there. Now that you understand all the mental and physical hardships involved and where the potential mine fields are in any weight-loss program, you're ready for a few practical tips to jumpstart your new life!

As you get started, you will learn a lot about what makes you tick. Many changes may be necessary in order for you to succeed. Some relate to your attitudes about food and eating. Others involve decisions regarding what is really important and how to prioritize the areas of your life. All of the changes depend on whether you are willing to take responsibility for the decisions you make and whether you can commit to yourself. There are also a number of more practical considerations that make losing weight easier. They might not be intuitive, but they were very helpful to the subjects who lost the most weight in the clinical trial. Here are a number of suggestions they incorporated into their routines.

1. Use a Logbook

Each participant in the study was provided with a spiral notebook that was small enough to be easily portable, but large enough in which to record daily observations, including food consumption, activities, stressors, sleep duration and quality, frustrations, questions, and suggestions. Dietary choices and activity levels are pillars of any weightloss program, and they were recorded assiduously. This diary was referred to as their logbook and was usually carried around in a purse, knapsack, or briefcase. It never left the side of each study volunteer.

When they initially enrolled in the study, many of the volunteers thought keeping a detailed record was a useless inconvenience. However, as the trial progressed, this perception changed dramatically. By the end they were all vocal supporters who praised the critical role the logbook had played in the success of the weight-loss process.

Although the participants personalized their logbooks and used them differently, each person recorded the key items that have been referred to in the program descriptions. On a daily basis they measured and listed the weights and amounts of everything they consumed. A typical entry, for example, might be:

- Salmon—4 ounces
- Asparagus stalks—6 with 1 pat of butter
- Garden salad—1-cups
- Oil and vinegar dressing with Italian seasoning—2 tsp.
- Salt and pepper
- Non-sweetened iced tea with 1 slice of lemon (12 ounces)

This level of detail is important in order for you to estimate the number of calories consumed or the fat-to-carb ratio. The logbook was also used to keep track of all activities. The subjects each wore pedometers that tallied the number of steps they took during the day as they went for walks, did chores around the house, ran up and down the stairs, or prepared meals. A similar approach was used for the resistance or weight-training portion of the activity regimen.

2. Prepare Food Beforehand

When you are really hungry, shopping for or preparing food doesn't make sense. That is when you are obsessing about what you can eat immediately. Invariably, in this scenario you are not going to make optimal food choices. You are more likely to select whatever can be wolfed down without preparation. It is best to undertake food preparation when you have sufficient time to plan and prepare high-quality snacks and meals. You can mix and match nutrient-dense, low-calorie choices in a creative fashion. Make munchies that are easily transported to work or that you can comfortably eat in the car when you are doing errands. Save those that are more appropriately kept in the refrigerator for home-based snacking. That way sugar, refined carbohydrates, and trans fats may be minimized, and your waistline will thank you.

Donald N swore by this approach. It prevented him from "going off the edge" many times. When he was able to eat some small healthy snack and wait for fifteen minutes, he wouldn't get hungry for hours. He now refers to this as his "fifteen minute" rule. It was so effective that many of the Biggest Losers adopted it.

3. Eat When You Are Hungry and Never Allow Yourself to Get Too Hungry

Many of our experts detailed what they snacked on when they began to feel hungry. The choices were as varied as the participants. Sammy J was a true believer in the celery and peanut butter approach. Michelle T swore by beef jerky, saying, "It was chewy, tasty, and expanded in my stomach." Kat N liked carrying around a mixture of almonds and pumpkin seeds with a few dried cranberries thrown in. "They provided a slightly salty sweetness that I loved. I ate a handful and felt satisfied for hours! They traveled well and stayed fresh for a long time. My coworkers even started doing the same thing. Remarkably, it helped several of them lose ten pounds!"

Marti B found success another way. "After you have crossed the line from realizing you need to eat to the real hunger zone, it's very difficult not to overeat once you start. You go from hanging on by your fingertips to an eating free fall." She went on to say that one thing that really helped was forgoing alcohol. "I must admit that I like a glass or two of wine with dinner. However, I frequently found that when I had something to drink it was harder to moderate what I ate. I guess my inhibitions were diminished when they needed to be even more discriminating. Alcohol also has a lot of calories! So cutting it out of my diet entirely was very helpful for me."

4. Your Pedometer Will Become Your Friend

"When I first saw my pedometer, I had no clue how it worked. I couldn't even turn it on. Once I figured out how to use it, I soon realized how inactive I was. It taught me a lot. When I finally became used to having it on my belt, I quickly learned how many steps I could add during the course of the day," said Maude F. This was a typical response from the study participants. "I never realized that little box could help me so much." And it did in several ways—not just by encouraging more steps per day (steps that could be added very easily while one was doing other necessary things without taking much additional time), but also by the curiosity and support it aroused in people who asked about it as they saw it being worn day after day. A number of participants' friends and coworkers even purchased one for themselves.

The fascinating thing that Trudy W noticed was that coworkers would ask, "How far have you walked today?" Or when she looked as if she was on her way to the snack machine, they would head her off and tell her she was doing so well losing weight that they didn't want her to take a step in the wrong direction. They actually became ardent supporters and saved her a number of times, reinforcing her willpower in the process.

5. Reading Labels Is Key!

"It's amazing what is hidden in foods to make them taste good. Who would have guessed they put high-fructose corn syrup in ketchup?" remarked Todd B. "What does that have to do with tomatoes?" Dottie was shocked that "partially hydrogenated sunflower oil is how trans fats appear on food labels. I knew they were bad, and although I checked every label for them, I didn't know that's what they were called in the food business. I guess they do it that way to pull the wool over our eyes."

Most of the participants said they really benefited from the label reading exercise. Almost uniformly they reported they were stunned by the hidden amount of salt and sugar in the food they brought home from the grocery store. They were surprised at all the seemingly "nonessential" ingredients such as flavoring agents, colors, and stabilizers contained in the groceries that filled their shopping carts. Whether you believe artificial sweeteners are safe or not, you need to be aware of where they are lurking so you can make informed decisions about what you put in your mouth. So remember the next time (and every time thereafter) you go shopping, READ THE LABELS!

6. A Treat Rather Than a Cheat

We are not on this planet very long. While some of us eat to live, most of us also live to eat. In real life we must determine how we organize our schedules, decide what to do, and choose how and what to eat. There are no food police looking over our shoulders. Nonetheless, we make many good decisions but also some that seem counterintuitive. Despite knowing what we should be eating, we often make different choices that might not appear to make sense. However, that is part of life, and a part that makes life worth living (the living to eat part)!

Jodie R had this perspective in mind when she remarked to the group, "I am calling this tiramisu a treat and not a cheat." What she meant by this was that she had built certain "indiscretions" into her eating approach so she didn't feel guilty when they occurred. She was well aware of what she was doing and made up for it by being scrupulous about what she ate both the day before and the day after. By treating herself for being "good," in her mind that dessert was not a cheat because it was planned for ahead of time. Other dietary choices were altered to appropriately incorporate the treat into her meal. So the best part was she didn't end up feeling guilty about what she had done.

7. Use a Scale to Monitor Portion Size

You may be surprised to learn that you're eating far larger portions than you realize. Initially, until you learn how to accurately estimate correct portion sizes, use measuring cups to dish out precisely two-thirds cup of carrots, one-quarter cup of almonds, or some other quantity of food, and buy a small scale to measure the weight of each piece of meat or fish. Shelly N's initial response had been that these extra steps were a colossal waste of time. Her daily schedule was already overbooked, and she literally found herself arriving late wherever she went. So it made no sense to her to unnecessarily complicate life further. That all changed, however, when she had to estimate an array of portion sizes in front of the other study participants. She soon found that her ability to "guesstimate" what comprised a half cup or a quarter pound was far from accurate. Not only was she frequently way off, she always overestimated, so her daily calorie intake was always about six to eight hundred calories more than she thought. This was a surprising yet very common finding among most of the study volunteers. This simple demonstration made Shelly a true believer in the utility of the food scale, especially once she learned that it required almost two hours of hard exercise to burn off all those extra calories she hadn't realized she was consuming. After using the measuring devices for four to six weeks,

Shelly realized she could make much more realistic estimates of her portion sizes. This insight accelerated her weight loss, and her renewed success made her even more motivated to stick with the program. She was not the only one to witness the power of such a simple intervention. What she found quite fascinating was both that she been eating 25 percent more calories than she had thought and that despite eventually eating less (after beginning to use her scale and measuring cups) she was not any hungrier.

8. Wine Is Permitted—Just Don't Overdo It!

Enjoy a glass of red or white wine with dinner. There is a correlation between light wine consumption and lower body weight. Wine contains healthy nutrients and makes most food taste better. However, I caution against excessive wine consumption because it isn't good for the brain, the heart, or the waist. As you pursue the activity program, compile your own weight-loss gems. That way, when you are queried about how you did it, you can easily pass along what worked for you.

Scott J. Barnard

CHAPTER 6

INTERMITTENT FASTING FOR WOMEN AND MEN

In a world that seems so desperate for answers about how to get rid of fat, we seem determined to overlook the most obvious solution: spend some time not eating. In my professional experience as a dietitian, and my personal experience experimenting myself with weight loss strategies I recommend for clients, intermittent fasting is a very efficient way to lose weight. It's also very good for your health, and saves you a great deal of both money and time. If you can exercise, all the better. Fasting for weight loss makes so much sense that it seems almost unnecessary to write a whole book on the subject.

Most of us actually believe that something bad will happen to our bodies if we fast—probably because we have absolutely zero experience with it. But fasting doesn't make you weak, tired, mentally cloudy, or any of the other things people worry about before they try it. Nor does it slow your metabolism—actually, it does the opposite of all these things, for reasons we'll explore in great detail in the sections ahead. Millions of people all over the world fast regularly as part of religious or cultural practices, and reap the benefits of improved physical health and emotional well-being.

But in our society, fasting is almost forbidden. The message we get again and again from nutrition author¬ities (not to mention every health and fitness magazine out there) is that the body needs small, frequent feedings throughout the day. Snacks are encouraged, and meals must never be skipped. As a result, we have literally convinced ourselves that we must eat all the time in order to avoid gaining weight. Does that really seem right to you? I find the idea absurd, and I think it has done a lot of harm to a lot of people. I suspect you're questioning it too, or else you wouldn't be ready to try intermittent fasting.

My goal in this book is to demonstrate to you that intermittent fasting is a very effective and safe way to lose weight—and specifically to lose body fat while retaining muscle mass. I aim to put to rest any fear you may have that skipping meals is bad for your body or will cause you to gain weight instead of lose it. I'll guide you with practical advice on how to integrate intermittent fasting into your life, and tips to make your fast go smoothly. I hope to have you so convinced of the benefits of fasting and the ease with which you can practice it that you commit to trying your first 24-hour fast before you finish this book.

If you've been fasting for a while then you already know that most people start out thinking they couldn't possibly do it and end up loving it so much that it becomes a permanent part of their life. If you haven't yet tried it and are worried about what it might be like (Won't I be hungry? Aren't we supposed to eat six meals a day? Can this possibly be good for me?), don't worry—by the end of the book you'll have read the personal stories of people just like you. People who thought they would never be able to go a day without eating, and who now practice all different styles of intermittent fasting that work with their busy schedules and life commitments—and keep them in the best physical shape of their adult lives. I believe you can start a fasting practice just as they did. If you are already a practiced intermittent faster and just want to expand your horizons, consider trying out a new fasting pattern while you read the book. With intermittent fasting, changing things up is encouraged.

I promote intermittent fasting because this strategy offers unique metabolic benefits that other "diet" regi-mens do not. I aim to show you in the parts ahead why that is so, and convince you that whatever "diet" you choose to follow or combination of foods you choose to eat, that intermittent fasting should be a corner-stone of your health maintenance plan. That said, I believe lot of solving the weight loss puzzle comes down to what works for you as an individual. In my experience, more of it is practical than metabolic. So I will ask you to keep an open mind. Not everyone loves fasting at first, but a lot of people who come to it believing it will be difficult find that it's actually quite enjoyable. Be willing to experiment a bit, and try some new ways to organize your eating habits. Because if you're trying to lose weight without too much fuss or deprivation, fasting sure is a nice tool to have in your toolbox.

More Than Just Ketosis

Ketosis is all the rage. Since you picked up this book, I'm guessing you're on the bandwagon. You're in good company here! Maybe you're on a ketogenic diet or considering it. And if you want to jump start ketosis, then intermittent fasting is your ticket. Truth be told, a ketogenic diet can be hard to maintain, simply because there are so many foods you can't eat. Even kale, the star vegetable of the 21st century, is only allowed in small amounts. I understand when clients say they're not up for the challenge of going keto. But I will tell you this: ketosis is divine.

Thankfully, if you don't want to do the ketogenic diet (or even if you do), there's a shortcut to ketosis—you can fast. Ketosis occurs when your body is burning ketones and fat for fuel instead of glucose. That happens in two situations: 1) no food is coming (fasting), or 2) few to no carbs are coming in (ketogenic dieting). When your body is in the fat-burning state, it makes lots of ketones in the process; hence, you are "in ketosis." It's completely normal for the body to be in ketosis, and it was certainly a common experience for humans throughout history who had intermittent access to food and periods of fasting in between. But the metabolic state of ketosis is very rare for anyone on a Western diet because (if I may speak for the crowd) we are always eating. When you're eating anything other than a ketogenic diet, you have effectively zero ketones in your blood. So it's quite uncommon for our generation of humans to be in a state of ketosis, unless you deliberately seek one out.

When you wake up in the morning after 8 hours of fasting, ketones levels are just beginning to rise. If you extend your fast until noon, ketone production will ramp up to supply some of the energy you need and your body will officially be in the famed fat-burning state of ketosis. Hooray! If you want to keep burning through body fat at a high rate, you need to stay in ketosis by sticking with your fast—for 16 or 24 hours, or a couple of days—and not by eating something ketogenic. There's a lot of attention on achieving ketosis with keto¬genic foods, but if you're consuming keto foods, then where do you think some of the ketones are coming from? Not the fat on your hips and thighs. Fasting for ketosis ensures that the ketones fueling your brain are coming only from your body fat, thus getting rid of it.

What Fasting Does for Your Body

Before we set our focus too narrowly on ketosis, let's consider the bigger picture. Yes, when you fast, fat will be burned and ketones will be made. But so much more happens when you're fasting—great things for the cells, tissues, and organs of your body, and some would say your mind and soul, too. If you have never fasted for even half a day in your life, then you may be thinking, "There's no way I can go 12 hours without eating!" But I am willing to bet that once you get started, you'll find it's a lot easier and way more fun than you ever thought possible, and you'll love it for a dozen reasons besides how quickly you'll lose your belly fat.

Fasting makes you burn through stored body fat when you haven't eaten for a while. You'll be burning so much fat that you'll be in ketosis. But fasting also trains your body to burn fat instead of glucose even when you're not fasting. In other words, fat burning isn't unique to the state of ketosis. Many cells in the body use fat all the time. The heart, muscles, liver, kidney, and other cells burn fat quite often. The trouble is that most of the time, while some fat is being burned, there's also new fat being made for storage because you're eating too much. Also, the cells that like to use fat rarely get the chance to do so for very long, because as soon as glucose comes in from a meal, they have to grab it instead. Too much glucose in the blood¬stream is toxic, so it can't be left sitting there. So the priority for cells is to burn glucose first, leaving the fat untouched.

Most cells in the body can use fat directly for energy, no ketones required. But if you've spent a lifetime eating six times a day and you don't exercise at all, then they probably won't be doing that, simply because they're out of practice and you're out of shape. But they can. And that is really the end game when it comes to intermittent fasting: losing fat and building muscle while improving your ability to use both fat and glucose efficiently.

The ability to switch between the two main energy sources and easily use either fuel when appropriate is known as metabolic flexibility. If your cells are healthy and already accustomed to burning fat when needed, then intermittent fasting will accelerate your fat burning and help you lose much more of it by forcing your body to rely on fat as its sole fuel source. This is what people are talking about when they say the ketogenic diet and intermittent fasting will turn you into a "fat-burning machine." If your cells are not metabolically healthy and have trouble using fat for energy, then you need to exercise to prime the fat-burning pathways in your cells. So as you may hear a lot around the intermittent fasting conversation, exercise is important not so much for the number of calories it burns but for the fact that it improves the ability of your cells to burn both glucose and fat when they are available or needed. Metabolic flexibility allows your body to use the food energy you give it, in whatever form, to actually provide your cells with energy—instead of using it to bulk up your fat stores and leaving you tired and hungry as a side effect.

When the metabolic machinery is working right—when you've been intermittently fasting and exercising for a while—you'll be better at burning fat anytime. And you don't necessarily need to be in ketosis for this to hap¬pen, although you'll accelerate the process if you spend a good amount of time there, as you do on a fast.

If cells can use fat directly for energy, what's the point of ketones? Ketones are made largely to protect against muscle wasting during a period without food, i.e., an extended fast. Here's why: the brain is not as metabolically flexible as the other organs, and it can't use fat. The brain uses glucose when it's around, and the brain uses a ton of energy. So what happens when we don't eat for a few days and glucose supply is tapped? It turns out that humans can make glucose inside our bodies and don't have to eat it at all. But we can only make a small amount, and it costs us some valuable amino acids from body protein (muscle) to do so. We don't want to lose muscle when we find ourselves without food for a few days, because that would weaken our arms and legs and other important functions our bodies deem necessary for survival. So the body developed the neat trick of turning body fat, stored just for this very purpose, into ketones for the brain, without sacrificing other important things.

Voila! Ketosis became the thing everyone's chasing, the holy grail of fat loss. We're on message boards boasting about beta-hydroxybutyrate levels and posting videos of ourselves drinking fat coffee in the morning to put us into nutritional ketosis before a workout—after which we may just go eat a normal meal. We have "keto bread" and "keto cookies" (anyone else getting flashbacks of SnackWells from the 1980s?), and if you don't ask too many questions, it's easy to conclude that as long as you're in ketosis, the fat is just melting away.

Is nutritional ketosis a marker that you're in a fat-burning state? Typically, yes. Does that mean you'll be skinnier next month? Maybe. But how much are you eating?

Ketosis Doesn't Always Equal Fat Loss

A person on a ketogenic diet can have high levels of ketones and never lose an ounce if they eat too much. Granted, overeating while in a state of ketosis is hard to do, because one of the benefits of ketones is that they significantly dampen your appetite. But people do it. And I don't care what mix of nutrients you're burning for energy; if you keep eating more than your body can use, you're not going to lose weight. In an attempt to trick the body into thinking we're fasting, a lot of us gorge on fat. But we never consider what ketosis is meant for in the first place. Our hunter-gatherer ancestors did not have stevia-sweetened fat bombs or bacon-wrapped, cheese-filled burger bites or MCT oil shakes when they were in ketosis. They were in ketosis because they just had no food.

The reason the term "ketosis" even appears on the cover of this book is because it's the one that you know to look for—and without it, you wouldn't know that this book is full of strategies to help you train your body to burn more fat. Am I a fan of ketosis? Yes! But I urge you not to chug ketone supplements and drink fat coffee all day and expect to shed pounds of fat. Being in a state of ketosis should mean that body fat from your belly, hips and thighs is providing most of the energy you need. However, if you're meeting all of your energy needs with keto foods you're consuming, then the body won't need to turn to your fat stores for anything at all. If you're careless, or overindulgent, you may net out on the positive side—storing more fat than you've burned!

If you're interested in ketosis and want to be sure that you're burning body fat instead of fat from your bacon breakfast, I recommend intermittent fasting. If you want to combine intermittent fasting and eat a ketogenic diet on the days you're eating, then go for it! Most of the recipes in this book can be used on a ketogenic diet, and we'll cover how to do it properly. Remember, you don't have to follow a ketogenic diet to achieve ketosis through fasting. But even if you do decide to go keto, don't skip the fasting part. That is the really good part—and it's likely to get you where you want to go faster.

The Unique Metabolic Benefits Of Intermittent Fasting

If you think about it for just a moment, you'll realize we're meant to fast intermittently. That's what body fat is for—to fuel your body when you're not eating.

But when are you not eating? We're taught to eat three meals a day with snacks in between, plus coffee or tea with sugar whenever we're in the mood (or worse, soda or juice with every meal), and, for some of us, wine, beer, or cocktails to round out the day. And that's just a normal Thursday. On special occasions, we go out to eat at a restaurant and consume double-sized portions, and surely, we eat dessert. We eat extra at celebrations (no one is ever too full for birthday cake), or because someone brought bagels to the office (even after we've had breakfast), or because we received a gift box of chocolate (so rude not to accept), or for any other reason that sounds good. And a few times a year, holiday meals make even restaurant portions look meager, as we firmly believe that holidays are for indulging in so much food that we joke about unbut¬toning our pants (or actually unbutton them) in order to sit comfortably after dinner.

Can you think of an occasion that calls for eating just a bit less in the same way holiday dinners give the green light to eat just a bit more? Ever heard of a holiday where everyone skips lunch? How about a national "underindulgence" day, where you take only small portions of food and leave some behind on your plate? If we have any of these, I haven't heard of them. I count the socially sanctioned occasions for abstaining from food to be the following: sleeping, taking a shower, using the bathroom, giving a presentation, and a few religious events. You might add "exercising" to the list, but I've seen enough people eat while exercising to disagree with you. We don't have nearly enough non-eating moments to balance out the eating moments. Most of our daily activities can be done while eating, and we proceed. We eat while working at our desk, driving to our destination, watching TV, relaxing at home, and so forth. We eat in between doing those things, if we feel like it. We simply don't take a break. If we snack after dinner and eat breakfast upon wak¬ing, our bodies get barely eight hours of rest from metabolizing food. All this overeating is making us sick, and there's no opportunity at all to balance it out—yet recommend that someone try fasting for weight loss and suddenly, you're an anarchist!

Of course, we know the nutrition party line. Eating small amounts at regular intervals throughout the day is the healthiest thing (so they say). It's not good for your body to go long periods without food (so they claim). You may have heard a number of arguments to support this recommendation, one of which is that you have to eat regularly to keep your blood sugar stable. This is absolutely untrue. The body has very tightly con¬trolled mechanisms for keeping blood sugar stable. In a healthy person, the concentration of glucose in the blood is about 5 grams, and will stay within a very narrow range whether they eat a giant piece of cake with 50 grams of sugar (10 times what's in the bloodstream already) or go three days without eating anything at all. Blood sugar does not drop abnormally low in a healthy person when they fast. Keeping blood sugar stable is simply not a legitimate reason to eat frequent meals.

The suggestion that frequent meals will help control blood sugar and prevent weight gain is a dangerous one, because it actually does the opposite. Eating releases insulin. In addition to helping cells take up sugar from the food you've eaten, insulin blocks the removal of fat from fat cells and prevents fat burning and body fat reduction. And the more often insulin is asked to do its job of getting glucose into cells, the less sen¬sitive cells become to its signal. Then, you have trouble using glucose for energy, and eating carbs further damages your health. We call that diabetes. But you also have high insulin levels, which means you'll have trouble using fat for energy, too, and you'll hold onto excess weight. This is how eating all the time breaks your metabolism.

A perfect solution to this problem is intermittent fasting. It undoes a lot of the harm that's been done from the frequent meals you've had all your life. Intermittent fasting prevents the constant stream of insulin from bombarding cells, and allows them to become sensitive again to its effects. Meanwhile, during your fast, as insulin levels fall, fats come out of fat cells and get burned for energy. This is how lowering insulin levels with fasting can produce weight loss, even in people who are insulin resistant, and prevent the progression toward diabetes or reverse the disease itself. We'll continue to explore the effects of fasting on insulin in the next section.

There are two other arguments in favor of the claim that eating all the time is a better approach than skip¬ping meals. The first is that fasting will put the body in "starvation mode" and slow your metabolism, causing you to gain weight instead of lose it. The second is that fasting will cause you to lose a great deal of muscle mass in addition to fat. These arguments raise good points about the risks of dieting, and we'll discuss below why these concerns are unfounded when it comes to intermittent fasting.

Low Insulin Levels Allow You to Burn Fat

When you eat, the pancreas releases insulin into the blood, and a domino effect occurs. Let's think about what was going on before first domino fell, when you were in the fasted state, such as while you were sleep¬ing. Upon waking up, your insulin levels would have been extremely low thanks to a long night of fasting. Fat from your fat cells would be fueling most of your body's energy needs, and you would just have begun to make ketones. If you waited a little longer to eat, then many tissues—including muscles, fat cells, and of course, the brain—would have been using them.

Then, you eat breakfast. Insulin levels almost immediately go up. Fats find their way back to your fat cells, along with some new ones coming in from the meal. They'll stay there for hours, until insulin levels drop again. What else is happening in the fed state? Assuming you've eaten some protein, the body will put those amino acids to use building new muscle, skin, or organ tissue, and other structures where they're needed. Assuming you've eaten some carbohydrate, glucose will be the body's main fuel source for the next one to four hours, and about a quarter of it will be stored in the liver and muscle for later use.

Insulin is what makes this all happen. It's the Head Hormone in Charge of energy use and storage. There are other players involved, but it's insulin that really runs the show. Insulin unlocks the door to cells and ushers glucose in. It grabs nutrients from the blood and stores them in fat cells. Assuming you've also eaten some fat with your breakfast, it takes three to four hours to be absorbed and stored away in your fat cells. This coincides nicely with the time that insulin levels (in a healthy person) take a good dive, meaning the hormone sticks around long enough to put away every last bit of food energy from your meal.

About six hours after eating, insulin levels return to baseline. You'd ideally move into the fasted state when insulin would stay low and the body would start to use fat for energy, keeping your weight nice and stable. But six hours of not eating? If you follow standard nutrition advice, you probably don't go half that long with¬out having a snack! Certainly, by six hours after a meal, you're usually sitting down for another meal. If your breakfast was at 8 a.m., lunch will likely be at 1 or 2 p.m., and dinner at 7 or 8 p.m. Just when fat storage is slowing down and the body is turning to fat for energy, chances are, you're going to eat again!

But let's assume you've caught on to the benefits of intermittent fasting, and you don't eat again six hours after your last meal. Now, insulin levels are low. It's no longer blocking the exit of fat from your fat cells, and you can start to burn it for energy. If you fast until breakfast the next day, you'll burn up lots of fat—most of it toward the end of your fast, while you're asleep.

The fat burning will keep going as long as you stay on your fast. Insulin will only rise again when you eat something. Since insulin is really the "gatekeeper" that allows fat in and out of your fat cells, then you have to avoid waking it up if you want to burn fat for energy. This is why "grazing" or snacking is terribly counter¬productive to weight loss. The goal is to keep insulin levels low and stay in the fasted state long enough to benefit from low insulin. While a 24-hour fast is great, you'll also get a lot of benefit from a 12 or 16 hour fast. If this seems way too much for you, don't worry. The hours add up faster than you think.

If you follow a ketogenic diet, then you may be wondering if all this applies to you. Fat, after all, doesn't cause an insulin response. The trouble is that even on a ketogenic diet, it's rarely the case that a meal contains pure fat. Even the most committed keto dieter doesn't eat pure butter or drink pure oil. Even bacon contains protein, as do other fatty meats, fish, eggs, and cheese. Nuts contain protein and carbs. Non-starchy vegetables like salad greens and broccoli contain carbs, too. So while the insulin spike from a ketogenic meal will be much lower than that of a typical meal, one shouldn't fool themselves into thinking there is no insulin at all. Two things to keep in mind if you are following a ketogenic diet and want to keep the insulin response low: 1) make sure not to eat too much protein, which triggers insulin release, and 2) do not "graze" all day on keto foods but rather keep distinct mealtimes, and extend your overnight fasting time before breakfast or after dinner.

Insulin Resistance and Weight Loss

Under normal circumstances, insulin levels should be low between meals and during a fast, and rise quickly to direct incoming nutrients to the right places when a meal is eaten. Then they should fall again to allow the body to burn fat between meals.

But what happens if insulin levels never go back down? This is exactly what happens in someone who is insulin resistant. In this case, the cells become resistant to the effects of insulin over time and the pancreas has to send out more and more insulin to get the cells to respond. Eventually, so much insulin is required to get the cells to respond that insulin levels never really go back down. They remain high between meals, and rise even higher when a meal is eaten. Insulin is a very powerful signal to the body to store fat, so a person with insulin resistance will have a very hard time burning fat and losing weight.

Why Does Insulin Resistance Develop?

When your body is bombarded with a lot of something, one of the ways it deals is by lowering its response to that thing. Someone who drinks a lot will become resistant to the effects of alcohol, and as time goes on, they'll be able to drink more and more before they feel the effects. Caffeine tolerance works this way, too. Maybe you used to have one cup in the morning and feel jittery, and now you have two, plus another in the afternoon, and tolerate them fine. Some drugs can produce the same effect. Resistance is a healthy defense the body has to protect from the harm of excess.

Of course, we don't always take the hint that the body needs us to stop giving it whatever it's resisting. The drinker may just drink more, risking damage to the liver and other organs. And while coffee has some excellent health benefits, the example is still instructive: coffee in the range of one to four cups a day is okay, but you do not want to get so tolerant to its effects that you're lurching from cup to cup all day long just to feel alert. That's exactly what happens when someone with insulin resistance eats multiple meals per day or grazes all day long. The cells are exposed to insulin with greater frequency, and they react by becoming even more resistant to it. This just makes the problem worse. Resistance is your body's way of telling you that's it had more than enough, and it needs a break.

What happens if we remove the thing that's causing the resistance? If the drinker quits drinking for a while, he'll notice that his tolerance for alcohol goes down, and it will take a lot less to feel the effects. If the all-day coffee drinker quits coffee for a month, she'll find that she has become much more sensitive to the effect of caffeine, and it'll only take one cup to do the trick. In other words, the body responds to the absence of something by becoming more sensitive to it. So, to solve the problem of insulin resistance, we have to essentially "quit" insulin. But how can you quit something that's made inside the body?

You can stop doing the thing that causes the body to make insulin in the first place: stop eating for a while. Insulin is only released after a meal. If you skip a meal (or many of them), you will reduce the amount of insu¬lin in your blood. Fasting is like a shut-off switch for the insulin production line in your pancreas: don't eat, and the machines stay turned off. Eat, and then eat and eat and eat more all day long, and the factory will be in full swing with no break in sight. In that case, insulin resistance will get worse, and when the body has finally had enough, it will progress to type 2 diabetes. In that case, the cells are so unwilling to respond to insulin that the pancreas cannot even make enough to force them to do so, and the person will need insu¬lin injections—supposedly for the rest of their life (they may not need insulin forever if they get into fasting therapy, but sadly, many diabetics aren't told about this option). Of course, taking insulin injections makes it nearly impossible to lose weight, since one of the big jobs of insulin is to store fat.

But you can absolutely prevent this from happening by fasting. Intermittent fasting shuts off the steady stream of insulin, lets cells become more sensitive to its effects, and reverses the progression to diabetes and a lifetime of weight gain.

Growth Hormone Reduces Fat and Increases Lean Mass

Growth hormone reduces body fat and increases bone and muscle mass growth. Hmm...get leaner, stron¬ger, and more resistant to osteoporosis later in life? How do I get this stuff?!

Growth hormone is, as you can imagine, very important in children because they are growing rapidly. We have less of it as we age, though it is still important, and is typically secreted during sleep. One of the func¬tions of growth hormone is to break down glycogen (the storage form of glucose) to release glucose into the bloodstream when energy is scarce. Fasting increases growth hormone, which, in addition to providing the body with energy, helps achieve the goal of losing fat while avoiding loss of muscle mass. A typical low-calorie weight loss diet (which most diets are) doesn't achieve the same result. It's for its muscle-build¬ing, fat-burning effect that you may have heard of bodybuilders using artificial growth hormone to get leaner and more muscular. But artificial hormones can cause unwanted health problems, sometimes quite serious, and taking them is a risky approach to improving one's physique. Luckily, intermittent fasting does it natu¬rally! Growth hormone, protein intake with your meals, and exercise help to preserve and build muscle mass.

Other things that stimulate the release of growth hormone are sleep (so it's good to get enough if you are seeking weight loss), exercise (ditto), and the "hunger hormone" ghrelin. Ghrelin is released to increase your appetite in the event that you skip a meal, and it also stimulates growth hormone. You'll notice it in bursts every so often when you're fasting. So when I'm fasting and I feel ghrelin telling me I'm hungry, I like to think that it's just there to tell growth hormone to build me nice strong muscles and bones, and I politely let it do its thing.

While new tissue is being built up by growth hormone, old tissues are also being broken down. But what happens to the old stuff? Good question! You see, the body does not keep all of its cells, proteins, cell membranes, and other parts forever. These things get old and worn out, and stop working properly. They need to be tossed out. In a sense, this is really what causes aging and disease— old parts piling up in cells and organs, clogging up all the machinery. Just as old knees and hip joints don't work as well as they used to, old liver and immune cells become defunct. So the body has mechanisms to clear out old parts that aren't working well and replace them with new ones, in an effort to keep things running smoothly.

One of the spectacular effects of fasting is autophagy (or "eating of self"), and it's the process whereby cells identify their own old and dysfunctional parts and destroy them, breaking down the structure and using whatever good parts are left behind to build something new and healthy. Suppose you have a smartphone that's glitching and you take it to the store to be fixed. You tell the technician that it freezes up when you open certain apps, the battery is draining too quickly, and the phone randomly shuts off for no reason. The technician uses some diagnostic equipment to identify which parts of the phone are broken, and then removes the old parts and installs new ones. The broken parts get disassembled even further, and perhaps the metal and electrical wiring that are still in good shape get transferred to a new battery whose other pieces were working well to begin with. Now it's got all the working parts.

Believe it or not, cells have that same ability to home in on what's broken and replace it with something new that works well, breaking down the broken pieces for energy when it's scarce and recycling the good parts to build new, properly working cellular components. But this process of autophagy is suppressed when a lot of new material in the form of nutrients is coming into the cell. In that scenario, there is pressure to build new components out of the materials coming in, and no time to devote to clearing out. So you are stuck with old parts as well as new ones, and things don't work as well as they could. During fasting, the body senses the absence of new nutrients coming in and triggers autophagy to begin the clearing out process so that, when you start eating again, there's a healthy foundation on which to build up new tissue. You can think of autoph¬agy kind of like spring cleaning: if you never go through your closet and get rid of clothes that no longer fit, then anything you buy will just be crammed in to the space available—but if you set time to get rid of the old stuff, everything new will fit nicely into the space you've created. The body's ability to focus on clearing out old and damaged proteins during a time of fasting does a lot of good things, including helping the immune system to work better, derailing the growth of cancer, and preventing the accumulation of fragmented pro¬teins in the brain that cause Alzheimer's disease.

So you can see how the combination of autophagy and increase in growth hormone really complement each other when you're fasting. Autophagy gets rid of out-of-date broken parts that are wearing the body down, and growth hormone builds up new tissues in their place. It's for this reason that growth hormone is reputed for its "anti-aging" effects.

The importance of growth hormone in maintaining muscle and bone mass and decreasing fat mass can be well understood from considering what happens when growth hormone levels are abnor¬mally low. Growth hormone deficiency is uncommon in adults and usually results from damage to the pituitary gland that produces growth hormone. Symptoms of this condition include a decrease in muscle size and strength, osteoporosis (a weakening of the bones), excess body fat (especially around the waist), and low energy levels—the opposite of what happens when growth hormone levels increase with intermittent fasting.

Intermittent Fasting And Your Metabolism

One of things most dreaded by dieters is the impact dieting has on the "speed" of their metabolism. (It's more relevant to consider energy expenditure, or how much energy you use that isn't formal exercise). When you eat less, as is the case with a low-calorie diet, you rob the body of some of the energy it's used to getting from food. To compensate, it uses less energy to perform basic functions such as metabolizing nutrients, maintaining body temperature, and so forth. The body conserves until energy going out matches food energy going in, and weight loss plateaus. If the person then decides to throw their diet out the window and increase the amount of food they eat, the body won't get the memo right away—instead, it will keep operating at a lower metabolic rate until it realizes that there is extra energy available and it can speed things up. But by that time, the person probably will have gained back all the weight they lost, and they'll be at square one.

Why does this happen? The body is smart, and it wants to match energy use with energy availability, lest things go haywire. Think about your computer. It requires electricity to power its processing activities. If you've ever been working at your computer and felt it get really hot, that was a sign that the machine was taking in too much energy and trying to get rid of excess by heating up. The body does the same. When too much energy comes in from food, it will speed up the metabolic rate by using more energy for its tasks, thereby getting rid of the extra it wasn't equipped to handle.

In contrast, say your computer is performing a lot of functions but isn't getting all the energy it needs. You're streaming a video online, you're trying to video chat with a friend, and your email program is open. The com¬puter can't access more energy to power all these tasks, and it doesn't want to shut any of them down, so it just reduces the energy supply to all of them. The video slows down and pauses a lot, your conversation is full of delays, and it takes forever for the sentence you're typing to appear in the email on your screen. That's what happens to the body, too. If you consistently give it less energy than it's used to, it uses less than it did before and it slows the whole machine down, thereby slowing down your metabolism or reducing your metabolic rate.

Intermittent fasting doesn't produce this same effect because you're not sending the body a consistent message that there's less energy to go around and it needs to conserve. You're sending alternating mes¬sages of no energy, then lots of energy. When there's no energy, the body takes what it needs from your fat stores. Before it has time to reduce energy output and slow metabolism, you eat the amount needed to satisfy your hunger and put fears of an energy shortage to rest—so there's no need for the body to slow the metabolism. Keep this in mind when you consider your fasting pattern: it's best to switch things up. If you choose the One Meal a Day pattern and eat the same number of calories day in and day out, your weight loss is more likely to plateau. If you're at your goal weight and just want maintenance, that's great! If you want to continue to lose, you may have to alter the pattern so that you vary between a lot of energy intake (an eating day) and little to no energy intake (one or more fasting days). When you eat, eat to satiety. That means you won't hold back or try to restrict calories when you're eating, but rather will eat as much as you need to feel comfortably satisfied with your meal. This alternating approach to fasting and eating normally has a very different effect on the body than a diet based on a consistent, rigid low-calorie daily budget. It doesn't allow for the body to settle in to a cycle of low energy intake and low energy expenditure, followed by weight plateau, which most dieters dread.

The release of adrenaline during fasting may also play a role in keeping the metabolic rate running high. Fasting, like exercise, is a mild stress on the body, and produces many of the same positive results—increased muscle mass, less fat, reduced inflammation, and so forth. The hormone adrenaline is released during times of stress, sending glucose and fats from storage out into the bloodstream to give you more energy (presumably to hunt and kill an animal for food, because your brain doesn't know we have grocery stores now). Depending on the person and the length of their fast, adrenaline can increase energy levels and may sometimes even interfere with sleep. The good news is, between the ketones helping you focus and the adrenaline giving you energy, you'll get a lot done.

How Is Intermittent Fasting Done?

I am willing to bet that you've already had experiences with intermittent fasting. Have you ever had a day at work that was so busy, the hours just flew by, and before you knew it, the day was nearly over and you'd had nothing to eat? Or, maybe you've taken a road trip and remember that despite being hungry, you held off grabbing snacks at the gas station so you could make it to your destination and have the appetite to eat a nice meal? Have you ever spent all day caring for a child and been so caught up attending to their needs that you forgot to feed yourself? If you've done any of these, then you've probably clocked 8, 9 or 10 hours fasting.

Fasting can be done in short bouts that can fit into your daily or weekly schedule and provide great benefits. It doesn't have to be a long, drawn out thing. "Intermittent" means to occur at irregular intervals, beginning and ending again without a continuous pattern. That's exactly what intermittent fasting is. You choose the periods of fasting and eating that work for you, and you can adjust them as you go. After you get comfortable with an intermittent fasting practice, you will create patterns that work for you.

Alternate-day fasting: Eat one day and fast the next day, alternating every day.

Intermittent fasting: Any combination of short periods of fasting. Some people do time-restricted eating every day and throw in one 36-hour fast per week on top of that. Some people fast on Monday, Wednesday, and Friday and eat freely Tuesday, Thursday, Saturday, and Sunday. You can do a three-day fast every other week. There are many patterns, such as a five-hour or even a one-hour daily eating window, fasting a few days per month, and so on. One of the best things about intermittent fasting is how flexible it is. Your goal is to alternate periods of eating with periods of not eating to elicit hormonal signals that tell your body to use stored fat for energy and keep your metabolic rate stable. You are encouraged to play around and adjust to find what works for you.

How The Body Gets Energy While Fasting

Any day of the year, whether you're fasting or feasting, the body gets energy from either glucose or fat. Amino acids from proteins can also provide energy, but since protein is so vital to body functions, there are many mechanisms in place to spare amino acids from being used for energy (one of which is the production of ketones, as you shall see in this section). In a healthy person who eats a typical diet of carbs, fats, and proteins, the body will primarily use glucose for energy during and after meals, and primarily fat when it has been a long time since a meal. A metabolically healthy person will swing back and forth between function¬ing on a glucose-based metabolism and a fat-based one, a lot like a hybrid vehicle that can be alternately powered by electricity or gasoline, depending on its mode of operation.

The main signal that tells the body which fuel source to use is insulin. In a healthy person, when insulin levels are high, the main fuel source will be glucose. When insulin levels are low, fat will take over as the main energy source. If you follow a ketogenic diet, then you should have persistently low insulin levels and your "car" will mostly run on fat, without switching over to the glucose fuel. But remember: that fat can come from either foods you eat or the fat you carry on your body, depending on how much you're eating. So if it's weight loss that you're after, don't add too much new fat to the existing supply! Spend some time fasting, even if you are following a ketogenic diet.

Since the human body needs energy all the time, regardless of whether food is available, it developed very good mechanisms for storing energy after food is taken in and later drawing on those storage depots when food is not available. For most of human history, food was much more scarce than it is today, and the body needed to use these stores a lot. Because of this ability to store food energy, we don't have to eat all the time. There's no physical need for a regular daily meal schedule. The default pattern of breakfast, lunch, and dinner is just something we made up! You have no obligation to follow it.

The body has specific storage depots for both glucose and fat. Glucose is only stored for short-term use, about a day or so. Fat storage, on the other hand, is apparently limitless. An average person can go some weeks without eating, relying exclusively on their body fat for energy. Someone with more fat can, as a gen¬eral rule, fast longer than a thin person if they have the water, vitamins, and minerals they need.

Glucose Storage

Glucose comes into the body when you eat any carbohydrate food. All carbohydrates, not just things we think of as sweets or starches, are eventually broken down to release glucose into the bloodstream. Broccoli, sweet potatoes, spinach, rice, chocolate chips, nectarines, lettuce, you name it—they all contain carbohydrates that will convert to glucose for energy metabolism. The pancreas releases insulin, which helps direct glucose to three places:

- to body cells, where it's used up for energy
- to the liver and muscles for short-term storage, and
- to be converted to fat and stored in fat cells for long-term use.

Glucose is stored in a chain called glycogen in the liver and muscles for the short term. A good amount of glycogen is stored in skeletal muscle for local use, but liver glycogen can supply energy for the rest of the body. You could think of liver glycogen like a candy necklace, where each little bead is one molecule of glu¬cose and the necklace can only fit 100 beads. When there is a need for glucose, as is the case a few hours after a meal, the liver pops off those sugary little beads one at a time to feed into the bloodstream, where they can travel to cells that need them. The next time you eat carbohydrates, new beads of glucose are strung onto the chain until it's full again, with 100 beads. Later, when it's been a while since you've eaten, the process of releasing the beads into the bloodstream is repeated, and the necklace is left half full. When you eat another meal containing carbohydrates, your glycogen stores are replenished again. And so on.

If you don't eat (or don't eat carbs) and the body dips into your glycogen stores, they will only last about a day. The brain is a big energy hog, and it gobbles up much of the glucose the liver sends out from glycogen. After one day of fasting, when you have depleted your glycogen stores, the brain still wants to be fed, and the body will have to turn elsewhere for its glucose supply.

Fat Storage

The body can't store very much food energy as glucose. But we must store it somehow, so of course, it is stored as fat! When we talk about fat being stored in the body, we are really referring to triglycerides. You have probably heard this term before when you had blood work done at an annual physical. Fat is stored in a triglyceride molecule, which has two parts: fatty acids, or what we'll refer to as "fat" for simplicity's sake, and another part called glycerol, which is actually used to make glucose inside the body. It's worth repeating that any extra energy in the diet is stored as fat. So, if you eat too much carbohydrate, you won't store it as glucose—after you've filled your glycogen stores—you'll turn it into fat and store it as triglycerides in your fat cells. Fat stores in your body will continue to grow as long as you continue to feed them!

When triglycerides come out of storage to be used for energy, they are broken down into fatty acids and glycerol, which are used in separate pathways for energy production. Glycerol is used to produce glucose, while some fatty acids are used directly by cells and some are converted into ketone bodies in the liver. So in addition to storing a large quantity of energy, fat stores are really quite diverse and can supply energy via three different types of molecules that serve the body's needs in different ways, as you'll see in the following pages.

How long could that magnificent storage depot feed you if you suddenly found yourself alone on a desert island without food? To put things in perspective, if an average 145-pound person has a body fat percent¬age between 15 and 30 percent, they will have 10 to 20 kg of body fat on them, averaging 15 kg (15,000 g). Fat provides energy at a rate of 9 calories per gram, so 9 cal x 15,000 g = 135,000 cal. That's two months' worth of energy! Compare that to one day's worth of glucose in storage and you can easily see that the body is designed to meet its long-term energy needs using fat. Eighty percent of the body's energy is stored as fat. The table below compares glucose and fat stores in the body.

Indeed, there are reports of people fasting for two months or longer under medical supervision to reduce significant obesity. But a prolonged fast is not something to take lightly. There is a tremen¬dous difference between the simple practice of fasting for 24 hours on alternating days and the complicated matter of going without food for weeks or months, which can be deadly.

So far, we have seen that there are stores of glucose and fat in the body, but the amount of fat far exceeds that of glucose. We know that over a long period of time without food, the body turns to fat for energy. But it's not quite as simple as that.

There are many different types of cells in the body, and they don't all have equal capacity to use fat or glucose as a fuel. Some cells are more flexible than others are. Cells in the heart, for instance, can use fat, ketones, and glucose. The cells in the brain and central nervous system prefer to use glucose, if it's available, or they can use ketones, but they can't use fat. Muscle cells can use fat, ketones, and glucose, depending on what's available and on what type of work the muscle is doing at the time.

So you can see that some cells are like the open-minded eaters in your group of friends—they'll have Italian, Mexican, Chinese, Thai, or anything else for dinner, depending on what's convenient. We want to convince more cells to be like these open-minded eaters and consider fat as a fuel source. That will help us achieve our goal of losing body fat.

The ability of your cells to use and easily switch between different fuels is called "metabolic flexibility." One of the goals of intermittent fasting is to improve metabolic flexibility. What affects metabolic flexibility? Some things you unfortunately can't change, like your genes, and how you've eaten and exercised all your life up to now. And some things you can change, like your level of fitness, your body composition, your stress and sleep levels, and how you choose to eat and exercise going forward.

The Body's Glucose Factory

Regardless of how metabolically flexible your system is, certain cells are not at all flexible when it comes to their energy source. These are like the picky eaters among your friends who always have to choose the restaurant and will take the whole group out of the way just to find the one thing they will eat. And this is where things start to get interesting when it comes to fat burning and ketosis.

Red blood cells, a part of the kidney called the renal medulla, certain cells in the eye, and some others can only use glucose for energy. And because we have no way to store glucose for long-term use (remember that the body has only about a day's worth of glycogen), we have to make our own glucose to feed these cells from the second day of fasting and beyond. Many people are surprised to find out that humans can make their own glucose! This flies in the face of the (bad) advice they have been getting that you have to eat carbohydrates every day to fuel the brain.The process of making new glucose is called gluconeogenesis— gluco for glucose, neo for new, and gen¬esis for creation. The ingredients for gluconeogenesis come from body fat, muscle tissue, and the recycled products of other metabolic processes. Only certain materials can be turned into glucose. Specifically, only the glycerol portion of a fat (triglyceride) molecule contributes to gluconeogenesis—the fatty acid portion gets used by cells that can use fat directly, or is converted to ketones for those that cannot. Certain amino acids, especially alanine and glutamine, are heavily relied upon to produce new glucose; these come from breakdown of muscle tissue and other means.

The body is very good at recycling nutrients. Muscle cells use the branched-chain amino acids valine, leucine, and isoleucine; conveniently, the process of breaking these down for energy releases alanine and glutamine, which are then diverted into glucose production. Lactate, released when muscle cells use glu¬cose for energy while doing certain types of work (you may be familiar with lactic acid, which causes the "burn" with muscle exercise), is essentially a waste product that's recycled to create new glucose. The red blood cells and the renal medulla that are so dependent on glucose also produce lactate in the process of using it, and so provide some of the raw materials for the production of the very nutrient they need to survive in a continuous cycle of reuse.

Ketones Solve Two Big Problems

Humans can starve for a period of time without our muscle tissue wasting away because we can produce ketones, which can provide energy to the brain. Remember, the brain uses about a fifth of the body's energy, and it's metabolically "expensive" to provide that amount of energy in the form of glucose made in part from amino acids. You might think, "Hmm, if only the brain could use fat like all the other organs, that would really solve our problems." And that's where ketones come in.

Ketones are made from fat, and the brain can use them as an alternative to glucose. Hooray! We've got lots of fat. Producing ketones is a way to make fat do more jobs in the body and get used up more quickly. This adaptation helps conserve body protein during prolonged periods without food. It's one of the reasons why muscle mass is not rapidly lost during a fast to provide amino acids for glucose production. I've heard some people say that they are worried about being in ketosis because the body "catabolizes body protein," i.e., breaks down muscle to produce ketones. That's not true. Ketone production "catabolizes" (or breaks down) fat, if you want to phrase it that way, and actually helps protect against breakdown of body protein.

Ketones are always being produced, but in such small amounts that they are barely detectable in the blood stream and make no meaningful contribution to the body's energy needs. An extended period of low insulin levels and dwindling glycogen stores will increase production of ketones to physiologically significant levels, and a fast that extends beyond the point of glycogen depletion will boost ketone production further. Ketosis begins at a low level, for most people, after an overnight fast. Individual differences in biology determine how quickly, and to what degree, ketosis occurs after some hours or days of fasting.

We can also look at this adaptation as a way to spare glucose for the tissues that really need it. In the fasted state, skeletal muscle will shift almost entirely to fatty acids for its energy needs. The brain shifts to using ketones for two-thirds of its energy. But the red blood cells and the renal medulla still need glucose, and they can be fed now with the smaller supply that is available.

So now you have an idea of what is happening in ketosis, and why a period of two to three days or longer without food can promote significant fat loss without simultaneously promoting rapid loss of muscle mass.

Ketone Testing

Ketones provide for less than 5 percent of the body's energy needs after an overnight fast, and about 30 to 40 percent of the body's energy needs after three days of fasting. As a fast progresses and more fat is burned for energy, the blood level of ketones rises. Consequently, many people are interested in testing their ketone levels to see how "deep into ketosis" they are and/or how fast they achieve ketosis.

There are three ketone bodies of interest: the first is acetoacetate (AcAc), which gets converted into two other ketones, 3-β-hydroxybutyrate (3HB) and acetone. Of these, 3HB is the ketone that circulates in the blood stream and provides the majority of ketone energy to the body.

There are also three types of testing to measure the three types of ketones. Urine strips are by far the most common testing tool of the average ketogenic dieter. They're inexpensive, easy to get at any pharmacy, and don't require pricking oneself with a needle. Unfortunately, urine ketone measurement doesn't accurately reflect ketone use in the body. Urine strips measure acetoacetate that is spilling out in the urine. The body is getting rid of ketones it can't use by excreting them in the urine. This isn't the goal! The goal is to use ketones for cellular energy. When cells are well adapted to using ketones for energy, the body retains the acetoacetate rather than wasting it in the urine. So, urine strips will generally show "less ketosis" (i.e., less wasting of ketones through the urine) as the body's ability to use ketones increases. Therefore, urine strips are unable to give any meaningful result—a high reading means the body is wasting ketones (not ideal), and a low reading either means you're not producing ketones in sufficient quantity to measure (i.e., you're not in ketosis), or that your body has become quite good at using ketones and has stopped excreting them in the urine (i.e., you're keto-adapted). Urine strips aren't very useful as a measuring tool.

Breath ketone detection devices measure acetone, which is excreted through the breath. This is probably the second most common measurement tool among keto dieters. Although a breathalyzer is more expensive than urine strips, it's only a one-time purchase (about $75 to $150). And no needle pricking is required for this method, either. Unfortunately, there is disagreement over whether breath ketone meters can give a reliable sense of blood ketone levels, and consistency of results is considered poor.

Blood ketone measurements are the most accurate but least convenient testing method. For those who really want to understand how different foods or types of exercise impact their ketone levels, or simply how ketone levels change with fasting time, then blood ketone testing of 3HB levels is the way to go. Blood testing requires pricking your finger with a needle and dropping blood onto a testing strip. It's also more expensive than the other two methods—a blood ketone testing meter for at-home use can be purchased for as little about $50, but the testing strips are pricey and the cost adds up over time. But if you're really curi¬ous about your how your metabolism is affected by your fast or a ketogenic diet, then it may be worth the inconvenience! A good level of ketosis will correlate for most people with a BHB level of 1.5 to 3.0 mmol/L. You can measure your blood ketones upon waking, after each meal or snack, and before bed. You'll be able to see how different foods and activities impact your blood ketone levels and can use that information to fine-tune your diet or fasting window.

Hunger And Satiety

Intermittent fasting gives you free reign to eat what and when you want as long as you're within your eating window. Still, it's worth embracing my number one rule for weight loss: if you're not hungry, don't eat. I don't care if it's dinner time. Your body doesn't seem to need food, so why feed it? Consider yourself lucky for the extra hour, and go do something else! Take a walk, call a friend, clean your house, organize your vacation photos—use the time for something other than adhering to a made-up meal schedule.

This urge to eat on a socially acceptable schedule is something we really buy into as adults. Children have a much better understanding of their physical need for food, and if you watch them, you'll notice they eat at irregular intervals, sometimes eating a lot, sometimes eating two bites or simply rejecting a meal outright (much to their parents' concern). Yes, they're growing, but that's not the only reason they eat that way. They are also better at responding to what they need and don't need when it comes to nourishment. Some very clever studies have shown that at the age of three, children are able to tell when they're full and stop eat¬ing, whereas by age six, children start to become as confused as adults about when to stop eating. They respond more to whether there is food in front of them than to whether they're hungry. They begin to eat more than they need, and they will probably do so for a lifetime.

But eating just because food is available or because it is a certain time of day is not the best strategy for weight loss. Feeling hungry sometimes is okay. No harm will come to you. But what makes us hungry any¬way? Is there anything we can do to lessen sensations of hunger when we diet?

How Hunger Works

Many factors contribute to a feeling of hunger and the desire to eat or stop eating. Internally, hormones released in response to nutrients from a meal signal that the body has had enough nutrition, which prompts us to put down to the fork. A drop in nutrient availability (as happens when it's been a while since a meal, or after intense exercise) will turn up the appetite, as will certain hormones released in response to circadian rhythm or nutrient balance. Externally, the smell of food or the sight of an appealing dish can make us start salivating, signaling the beginnings of digestion and the body's anticipation of food to come. After you've eaten a lot, these same sights and smells might make you feel a little queasy, reminding you that fullness or satiety is just as real a sensation as hunger.

Growth hormone, helps break down and get rid of body fat and build up muscle tissue. So if you can stick with your fast and ride one or two waves of a ghrelin peak, some very good things will happen!

If you choose to respond to ghrelin by eating, your fast will be broken, insulin levels will rise, and you won't start burning body fat again until a few hours after your meal. The option to eat is always available to you, though you often won't take it. Above all, be sure that you take good care of yourself and allow some flex¬ibility in your fasting practice. Some days you'll be more interested in going longer before eating—or more likely, you'll just be busier and won't really notice the hunger, which is why one of the tricks to fasting suc¬cessfully is to keep busy. Other days, you'll hear ghrelin shouting at you and you will choose to eat so that it quiets down. And that's perfectly fine. Fasting should be challenging and push you to be more flexible with your eating habits. But it should not be so uncomfortable that you're miserable. You're trying to develop a new habit that you can stick with for a lifetime—and no one would keep up with something that makes them miserable.

Leptin, a Satiety Hormone

The whole story of how the body receives hunger and satiety signals is complex, and better suited to an endocrinology textbook. So we'll just get acquainted with one more celebrity hormone before we move on.You may have heard of the hormone leptin, secreted by fat cells, which sends signals to the brain about the size of the body's fat stores to help regulate appetite and energy expenditure. People with more fat have more leptin. If all is working as it should, an overweight person will secrete a lot of leptin, which will reduce their appetite and make their body use more energy, thereby reducing the size of their fat stores and restoring balance to the system. But things can go awry if a person has much too much fat and leptin. In that scenario, the brain becomes resistant to leptin's signals and the person doesn't get the message to eat less; as they continue to eat and store more fat, the fat cells produce more leptin, which just makes the whole problem worse. This is called leptin resistance, and it's similar to the problem of insulin resistance. People who are leptin resistant won't get the benefit of a reduced appetite that leptin should provide, because the system is broken. Losing some body fat will reduce leptin levels and allow the brain to become re-sensitized to it.

Other Contributing Factors

Ghrelin isn't the only thing that makes us hungry, and leptin isn't the only thing that tells us to stop eating. There are many hormones that influence hunger and satiety, and other mechanisms in the body for regu-lating food intake. For instance, peptide YY is a hormone released from the small intestine in proportional response to food intake (more food, more peptide YY). It slows the movement of food through the digestive tract and binds to receptors in the brain that make you feel full. Like other hormones, it peaks and falls: levels are highest in the second hour after a meal and fall steadily thereafter.

In addition to hormones, there are other physiologic cues that adequate food has been eaten, or that more food is needed. For instance, certain sensors in the lining of the stomach stretch when food is eaten to sig-nal the brain to decrease appetite. Foods and beverages that cause expansion of the stomach work through this mechanism to create satiety. This is one of the ways that fiber, which expands to absorb water in the digestive tract, helps to create a sense of fullness. Another trick sometimes used by people who fast is to drink lots of water to expand their belly if they want to prevent hunger. Deficiency or insufficiency of micro-nutrients can increase hunger and food intake. You can avoid this by eating a nutritious diet that provides adequate vitamins and minerals, or by taking a supplement to fill in any gaps if you feel your diet is falling short.

It's interesting to realize that even though the body has such sophisticated mechanisms for controlling food intake to match its energy needs, hunger levels go way down after a couple of days of fasting, when we would imagine nutrients are sorely needed. Ghrelin levels peak on day 2 of a fast and steadily decline thereafter, allowing hunger and the desire to eat to subside. Ketones, present in significantly higher amounts after two days of fasting, dampen the appetite as well. A conclusion can be drawn that a few days of fasting doesn't rob the body of nourishment that it needs, and that short periods of fasting are not harmful. If the body was starving, it would use all the tools it has—notably, ghrelin and the sensation of hunger—to make you uncomfortable and persuade you to eat. But the opposite is true: most people feel very well after a couple of days of fasting and don't really have a desire to eat.

It's Good to Skip Meals!

I hope I have convinced you by now that it's okay to skip meals. If you want to avoid gaining weight, it's a good idea not to eat when you're not hungry. If you're overweight, skipping meals when you're not hungry is a no-brainer. Skipping meals when you are hungry is a bit harder, but I imagine you've done much harder things in your life and I have no doubt you can do this too. If you can give yourself permission to set aside the hunger until it dissipates instead of reaching for a snack, and you can do that through breakfast and lunch twice a week, then you'll be intermittent fasting for 48 hours each week! That's 48 hours that you'll give your body to burn through your fat stores, helping you lose the extra weight you're carrying. That's a really good thing!

If I haven't convinced you by now that the body can thrive without three meals a day, I think I may know why. It's breakfast, isn't it? You have heard all your life that no matter what, you must not skip breakfast. Breakfast can be the last holdout. I hope you can believe me when I say that eating breakfast will not make you a healthier person. And moreover, eating before the hour of 9 a.m. does not magically make you lose weight. Eating breakfast is not the nutritional equivalent of doing three high-intensity interval workouts a week. It offers no special advantage to your metabolic health. It's just a meal eaten in the morning—and one that most Americans can't manage to consume without a day's worth of sugar. If you are actually hungry when you wake up in the morning, then go ahead and eat breakfast. Choose something high quality that's rich in protein and/or fat, with no sugar or flour. But if you are someone who does not get hungry in the morning, consider yourself lucky! You've been granted a free pass and can sidestep the nutritional landmine that is Breakfast in America. Please, for heaven's sake, skip it. Skipping breakfast will not do you harm.

Don't believe me? Then believe Mark Mattson. A 2016 article in The New York Times titled "Fasting Diets Are Gaining Acceptance" said this about Mark: "Mark Mattson, a neuroscientist at the National Institute on Aging in Maryland, has not had breakfast in 35 years. Most days he practices a form of fasting—skipping lunch, taking a midafternoon run, and then eating all of his daily calories (about 2,000) in a six-hour window starting in the afternoon." Mark Mattson has devoted his entire professional life to the study of healthy aging at the biggest health research organization in the country. If he thinks skipping breakfast is such a good idea that he's been doing it for 35 years, then maybe the rest of us should get on board.

Metabolic Flexibility And Using More Energy

If your cells are not already well-equipped to use fat for fuel, then in order to take full advantage of the fat burning benefits of intermittent fasting, you need to help your cells become more metabolically flexible.

Your body has many specialized cells, such as red blood cells, brain cells, and muscle cells, each of which need energy to do their cellular work. For example, liver cells work to detoxify substances that come into the body and kidney cells work to filter the blood and create urine. Most of the energy your body uses in a given day powers these functions, which are the minimum processes needed to keep your body alive and well. The sum total of all the energy needed for these minimum required tasks is called Resting Energy Expenditure, or REE. This energy comes from the macronutrients—carbohydrates, fats, and to a lesser extent, protein or amino acids (though, as discussed previously, protein contributes relatively little to the body's energy needs because it is needed for other things).

What Is Metabolic Flexibility?

For the purpose of providing energy to cells, carbs are broken down into glucose, and fats are broken down into fatty acids (and later ketones). Fat and glucose are the major fuel sources, and many cells can make use of either depending on what's available and what is needed at the time. Muscle cells, for instance, want to use fats while at rest, and glucose when they're contracting, such as during exercise. In a healthy person, these cells will be able to shift back and forth between the fuels as the situation demands, and get energy from either one without difficulty. But this is not always the case. With poor eating and sleep habits and lack of exercise, the cells can become metabolically inflexible—meaning they can't use the different fuels very well, or switch back and forth between them. The classic case of this is someone with diabetes: they can't use glucose very well, so it remains in their bloodstream and promotes weight gain due to persistently high insulin levels.

What makes a healthy cell choose one fuel over another? It depends on a number of factors, including:

Availability: Are you fasting and have only fat as an energy source? Or did you just eat a high-carb meal and deliver a lot of glucose to your bloodstream?

Familiarity: Have you been eating only carb-heavy meals your whole life, and snacking constantly? Have you been on a ketogenic diet and/or intermittent fasting for a long while? This will impact the expression of genes and the concentration of compounds needed to metabolize glucose or fat.

Fitness of cells: What is the ability of your cells to extract energy from either fat or glucose? This is depen¬dent in part on your overall fitness level, which is influenced by the type of exercise you do, as well as genetics.

It is essential to maintain your metabolic flexibility. Without it, you are much more likely to gain weight or have trouble losing it, suffer from lack of energy, and eventually develop diabetes. We want our cells to be able to easily use fats for energy when we are fasting, or when the muscles are at rest (e.g., sitting or sleep¬ing). And we want the cells to be able to use glucose easily for energy when a meal delivers glucose to the bloodstream, or when the muscles are doing intense work (e.g., sprinting, lifting a heavy weight).

Using More Energy

In addition to making sure cells can easily use the energy you give them from fat or glucose, you also want to take steps to increase the amount of energy you use overall—i.e., your energy expenditure. Remember, extra energy from food you eat is stored as fat. The more energy you use, the less you will carry around with you. So how can you use more energy?

An important concern for someone on a weight loss diet is that it will slow down their metabolism, which over time will cause them to plateau and regain the weight. This is hugely important and should not be overlooked! We know that we not only want to lose weight, but also want to keep it off. One of the benefits of fasting for weight loss or maintenance is that fasting prompts release of the hormone adrenaline, which increases the metabolic rate. This is in contrast to a calorie-restricted diet, which tends to decrease the metabolic rate.

What do people actually mean when they say that dieting slows your metabolism or decreases your metabolic rate? They are really talking about the body's ability to reduce the amount of energy it uses in a given day, i.e., Total Daily Energy Expenditure (TDEE). The amount of energy the body spends in a day is dependent on a number of factors, including: age, gender, the type and amount of food you eat, and the amount of muscle mass you carry on your body. It's also dependent on how much you move around, irrespective of how much "formal exercise" (e.g., hours on the elliptical machine) you do. Movement itself is key to using more energy.

Many people know that muscle mass uses more energy than fat mass, regardless of exercise regimen. Of course, it's exercise that maintains muscle mass in the first place! And some people worry about losing muscle when they diet. We have already seen that growth hormone triggered by intermittent fasting helps build muscle mass. It's also worth noting that we don't have to sit around and "worry" about losing muscle when we lose weight—we can actually get up and grow some more! Muscles get bigger when your body is convinced it needs bigger muscles to do more work. So, lift some heavy things, start including strength training in your exercise plan, and grow some bigger muscles.

Keep Your Metabolic Rate High: Get Moving

Maybe you know that movement is important to maintaining weight loss, but you don't have an exercise routine or you have struggled to start one. A lot of people are in your shoes, and there are smart ways to get started and keep going. I believe there are two main barriers that keep people from getting enough move¬ment or exercise: The first is perceived lack of time, and the second is that they haven't found any activities they really enjoy.

- Finding Time to Exercise

Whenever I start working with someone who tells me they don't exercise or just barely do so because they are just too busy, I have them do a couple of things to assess how they spend and perceive their time. I ask what percentage of their time they realistically feel they can devote to exercise now that weight loss is a pri¬ority for them. Most people tell me around 10 percent. To which I usually raise my eyebrows and say, "Wow! You're going to start doing 17 hours of exercise per week? That is really a lot!"

There are 168 hours in a week. Ten percent works out to 16.8 hours—way too much time to spend doing formal exercise. So I ask the busy people who are starting with zero hours of exercise per week to be a little more modest, and devote just 1 percent of their time to physical activity. That's 1.68 hours, or one hour and 45 minutes per week. This really puts in perspective how little you need to do to make an impact on your health and weight loss. Even the busiest of people find a way to do that.

If this sounds like you, take a piece of paper and track how you spend all 168 hours one week. List the days of the week at the top, and the activities—sleep, work, commuting, house chores, TV watching, time with family—on the side. Then just spend 2 minutes at the end of the day jotting down the number of hours you spend in each activity. After one week, many people find they've spent a dozen hours doing unimportant things. They come back and tell me they can easily double their exercise time to three hours per week. This person will spend one less hour on housework and two hours less watching TV, and they'll have three hours to exercise. By session two, we nip the "no time to exercise" problem in the bud!

Another interesting discovery on these time logs is the number of hours people spend preparing and con¬suming food. One of the great benefits of intermittent fasting, as I've mentioned before, is the enormous amount of time you'll save! If you currently cook your meals, you know it takes many hours every week to go to the grocery store, prep, cook, and of course, eat. Going out to dinner can be a two-hour affair. When you fast, you cut out multiple meals from your week and save a ton of time.

If you're someone who can't find the time to exercise, I recommend you try doing a weekly time log. It may be eye opening! If you haven't yet started your fasting schedule, consider doing a baseline time log and another a month or two after you've gotten into your fasting schedule—you may see significant time savings in the "food prep and eating" column.

- Finding "Exercise" That You Enjoy

Not surprisingly, not everyone loves lifting weights or spending an hour on the elliptical machine. But you may think you're supposed to exercise this way, because those are the things that are readily available to most of us though fitness gyms. As you've learned from the experts interviewed in this section, cardio machines are not the optimal path to weight loss and metabolic health! The best way to build muscles, prevent weight gain, and maintain your metabolic health is through regular movement of varying kinds. It does not have to be unappealing or excruciatingly difficult. It certainly should not be those things, or else you won't do it! It's best to find ways to move more in your daily life. Sprint to the bus stop, lift heavy rocks to clean up your backyard, play a round of basketball at the local park, dance to the tune of your favorite song, walk or bike anywhere you need to go—just get up and get moving while doing something that matters to you. Then, you are very likely to keep doing it.

A few years ago, I came across a study that made this point quite nicely. The study separated participants into two groups, gave all participants books to read, and tracked how often everyone went to the gym. The only difference between the groups was that the participants in one group had to leave their books at the gym and could only read while they were there, whereas participants in the other group could take their books home with them to read whenever they wanted. Who do you think went to the gym more? You guessed it: the people who left their books at the gym. They were willing to exercise more often in order to find out how the story would unfold! This drives home the point that attaching movement to something else that's important to you will increase the likelihood that you'll do it.

One of the best examples I've seen of this is when a married person who wants to spend more time exercis¬ing convinces their spouse to take a brisk nightly walk as part of their quality time together. Sometimes this is instead of or in addition to spending evening time on the couch in front of the TV. The benefit to the cou¬ple is that they both get healthy movement in their day, and they get quality time to talk and connect during their walk. It also eliminates the problem of deciding whether the gym is more important than time with your spouse! Some people make similar changes to interact in a physically active way with their children. They're motivated by the idea of quality time with those they love, so they play catch with the kids in the yard, or have a family run with the dog.

Other things may motivate you. If you want to make new friends, maybe an exercise class or yoga class is right for you. You might find a sports team you can join. If you like to contribute to a good cause, then you can easily find a charity that has training teams in your area for an annual fundraising event—for instance, you can train for a 5k to raise money for breast cancer research. Or volunteer to do something that requires movement instead of sitting still. I once volunteered for a day with Habitat for Humanity, an organization that builds houses for people in need of them. I was assigned to paint doors. Others were putting together house frames, and I thought I was getting off easy. Boy was I wrong! After a day of painting doors, my shoulders and biceps were so sore, I felt like I had done hours of weight lifting in the gym. But I dislike lifting weights, and I never would have done that much work in a gym environment. The experience of being with others contributing to a good cause was much more motivating to me, and I was happy to do it!

If you enjoy being in the outdoors, start doing activities outside. Hiking, biking, find a workout class in the park. Are there trails near your home that you've always wanted to explore? Grab a friend and take a bike or hike. Find a hill or inclined street in your neighborhood that looks like it would be a challenge to climb, and walk that direction. Do you find yourself driving to pick up your kids at a friend's home five minutes away? Walk there instead, and walk home with your kids so they can see a model of daily movement and grow up to value that in their own lives.

How To Get Started If You're Unsure

If you have never tried to fast for any amount of time and can't imagine even skipping a meal—let alone a whole day of eating—then I invite you to take a deep breath and remember that you don't have to jump in with both feet. There are dozens of relatively easy things you can do to lower the psychological barrier to fasting. That's what this section is all about. Of course, if you're a "dive right in" kind of person and want to get going, then by all means, get to it! There is no special preparation needed to begin fasting. You can start now.

Group your eating moments—don't graze: First and foremost, distinguish mealtimes from all other times. You can eat any amount of food you want—just eat it at either breakfast, lunch, or dinner. Respect that all other times are non-eating times. If you want dessert after dinner, eat it in the same "eating moment" as dinner itself. Don't get up, clear the table, wash the dishes, retire to the couch for a movie, and then eat dessert.

Similarly, don't nibble before breakfast, or have a mid-morning snack after breakfast. If you are hungry before and after breakfast, make yourself a bigger breakfast. And if you normally have a snack a couple hours after lunch, add that snack to the end of your lunch. Then, wait to eat again until dinner.

Swap heavy cream for sugar in your coffee or tea, or take it plain: This is a small but significant move. Many of us drink coffee or tea once or more per day. The beverages themselves have great health benefits, and I generally don't see reason to restrict them. The trouble comes when you add sugar or other sweet-eners to these beverages. They become just another source of sugar in our daily diets, and continue to reinforce the sugar cravings you are trying to put to rest. Instead of sugar, learn to take your coffee black and your tea plain. If you can't take it black, add heavy cream (not milk) or coconut oil or cinnamon if you like those flavors. Don't add almond milk or similar products that have carbohydrates, alternative sweeteners, or both. If you are fasting and want to take coffee or tea on your fasting day, it's helpful to get this practice under your belt.

Create a "no eating" buffer around your sleep time: If you're doing well with three meals a day and you aren't grazing or snacking in between, the next step is to create a mini "no eating" window after dinner and before breakfast. If you think about it, sleep is the longest period of fasting that most of us have every day—a nice eight hours or so. If you can push your first morning bite out two hours into the day, and make sure dinner wraps up two hours before bedtime, then you'll increase that fasting window by 50 percent! That's a fast of 12 hours, and is a real accomplishment. If this works for you, keep going that way, maybe pushing breakfast out two more hours the following week. You'll see that you may get to a 16-hour fast in no time.

Ask others about their fasting experiences: Fear of the unknown is one of the biggest challenges when it comes to fasting. For most of us who were raised in Western society, fasting is just not part of our culture. Its unfamiliarity makes it that much more intimidating.

So, don't venture into the great unknown all by yourself! Ask around your circles and find out who has a fast-ing practice, whether for weight loss, health, religious, or other reasons. They will have great advice to offer, and will be able to allay some of your fears. There are hundreds of groups and support circles out there. I am confident that you will find people in your social spheres who practice fasting, too. Personally, when I was looking to interview people about their fasting practices for this book, I simply asked around. I was surprised to learn that quite a few of my colleagues have a fasting practice, as well as a cousin of mine, and even some friends who work in the restaurant industry (not usually a place you find people turning down food!). So go find support to get started, and stay involved for the motivation to continue. There's nothing that helps a new habit stick better than being around others who practice the same.

Find a friend or family member who wants to try intermittent fasting with you: If you're not interested in asking far and wide and would rather have support closer to home, convince a family member or friend to try out a fasting practice with you. Preferably someone you share meals with, so you can organize the fast around your meal schedule and either do something else together during mealtimes, or break your fast together if the time is right. Maybe your spouse or partner is willing to do it, and you can both skip eating throughout the day, then come home to share a nice dinner together. Or maybe you have a coworker who wants to skip breakfast and lunch with you, and the two of you can take a quick walk on your lunch break instead of eating with the rest of the staff.

Finding a fasting partner not only creates accountability (you'll worry about letting them down if you "cheat"), but also a sense of companionship, someone to troubleshoot with and with whom to marvel at how easy it is after all. You'll feel you're not alone in the experience, that you have someone to call on who "gets it." In some ways, the gratification of sharing the experience may even be one of the things that motivates you to keep doing it.

Stop eating before your workout because you think you need the energy: Quit having a snack or energy drink or smoothie before a workout. If you exercise in the morning, experiment with a fasted workout. Make sure to drink water. You are likely to be just fine. If you're tentative about skipping the pre-workout snack, just take it a little slower than usual. The worst that could happen is you don't feel great afterward, so you take it easy and eat a meal and recover. But more likely, you will feel okay to try it again the next day.

That said, please use common sense: If you are very out of shape, haven't exercised in a year, and have never gone a few hours without eating in your entire life, don't just jump in and do a big workout in the mid-dle of your first fast! That's when you are likely to feel unwell. If you're just starting to exercise and starting to work your fasting muscle, set off by doing 10 minutes of exercise in the fasted state, and if that goes well, up it to 20. Be mindful of your own limits.

Stop saying "I have to eat": One thing that fasting teaches is that eating is a choice. For many of us, we were raised with people saying how much we "have to" eat at the dinner table. Society tells us we "have to" eat three meals a day, or a friend tells us we "have to" eat if it's been some number of hours since our last meal. Ever wonder how they know when your body needs food? Or how about being told you "have to" eat when you're sick and can't stomach any food? Presumably this is to "keep up your energy" while you're fighting off the illness. Has it ever occurred to these advice-givers that the energy required to metabolize your meal might indeed be better spent fighting off that very illness? People don't need food for all these arbitrary reasons. Once you get out of the habit of feeding the body simply to ease your emotional distress or the inflated concerns of those around you, then you will begin to see that the "have to eat" moments are really few and far between. Most of the time you are simply choos¬ing to eat to avoid an uncomfortable situation. It's certainly your right to make that choice. Just know it's a choice, not a necessity. And perhaps start saying to yourself, "I'll eat now because it feels right for this situation, but I don't actually have to." Over time, if you're not achieving the results you want, you may decide that it's not worth it.

Give your meal your full attention: Since you will have distinct mealtimes and won't be mindlessly nibbling throughout the day, devote your full attention to your meal when you have one. And now that you've stopped believing eating is something you "have to" do at any given time, you may feel more empowered when making the choice to devote some of your precious time to eating. Revel in your own authority. Mark the transition from whatever else you're doing to the occasion of eating a meal. Don't drive, read, or work at the computer while you're eating. If you have only 10 minutes, take the 10 minutes to stop whatever else you're doing and just eat. Sit down to your meal without distraction. You will appreciate the experience more, and you will begin to approach food will more consideration.

Cut way down on sugar: You may notice that eating sugar causes your appetite to swing wildly, which can make it more difficult to go from one meal to the next without snacking. Since we want to avoid snacking, sugar is not on our side. It also undermines the great progress you make when you stop believing you have to eat and become the master of your own eating habits instead. I am generally pessimistic about some¬one's prospects for significant weight loss and weight maintenance if they have an attachment to sugary foods. Things like soda, juice, sweetened drinks, cookies, candies, cakes, ice cream, "food bars," muffins, chocolate-covered things, pastries, sweetened crackers, dessert tarts made with coconut sugar and other "healthy sweeteners," dried fruit—the list never ends. Intermittent fasting can be quite difficult if you eat these foods on a regular basis. Long-term health outcomes are likely to be poor. Sugar in the amounts we consume it is flat-out dangerous. It's best to cut it way down, or cut it out.

The good news is, sugar cravings go away rather quickly when you stop feeding them. I generally ask clients who want to stop eating sugar to commit to seven days with no sweets at all, and a reassessment at that time to decide if they want to extend their sugar fast. The first week is usually the hardest, so by day 7, it hardly seems worth throwing away all that good work, and they recommit to seven more days. If sweets have a hold on you, I recommend trying seven days of no sweets or, if that seems unrealistic, try seven days during which you'll only eat something sweet once per day. After that, you can pick a few days to have a sweet thing, and a few days to skip it. You can decide where you want to go from there. Life without attach¬ment to sugar is better. It's a lot like life after quitting smoking. I've never heard anyone say they wish they still smoked. Ask someone who's kicked their sugar habit to tell you about it, and see for yourself.

Start eating more fat: Fat makes meals more satisfying so you can go longer between meals. Skip any¬thing labeled "low-fat." Instead, use full-fat dressings on salads and eat full-fat cheese or yogurt. Add sliced avocado to any dish. Use tahini (a sauce made from sesame seeds) as a dip or sauce for vegetables. Eat a handful of nuts with a meal that isn't very high in fat to begin with. If you eat breakfast and enjoy eggs, always have the yolk (don't just eat the whites), and have bacon on the side. Cook vegetables in a good amount of coconut oil or olive oil. If you take cream in your coffee, make sure it's heavy cream and not milk. Experiment with fat coffee or "bulletproof" coffee: blend 1 or 2 cups of black coffee with 1 tablespoon of butter and 1 tablespoon of coconut oil for a frothy, creamy mixture to drink in place of a meal. It's quite filling and energizing.

Observe your current eating patterns to see where you can easily stick in a fast: Take a few days to pay close attention to when you eat. What's the first thing you put in your mouth after you wake up? Is it coffee or tea, breakfast food, or water? Or do you busy yourself getting ready for work and run out the door, grabbing a breakfast sandwich on the way? Maybe you eat nothing at all in the morning. Whatever it is, just take note of your pattern.

Do the same for moments later in the day. When do you eat lunch, or do you skip it on busy days? What are your snacking habits? Is dinner a family affair that happens around the same time every night, or is your schedule more irregular, with late dinners on some evenings and early ones on others? You may discover that you already go long periods without eating, and that a bout of intermittent fasting here and there would not be a huge change from your normal routine. Many people tell me they don't eat breakfast anyway and usually eat lunch around noon. It's within reach for them to stop putting sugar in their morning coffee (this is probably harder than not eating, actually, but you can do it in a week), and quit snacking after dinner the night before, so they can achieve a 16-hour daily fasting window. Some people say that a certain day of the week is just chaos for them, and eating is impossible anyway. Do you have any days like this? Grab that opportunity!

Observe your hunger patterns: While you're observing your eating patterns, take careful stock of when you are hungry. Start by asking yourself if you're hungry in the moments before eating something, and note how soon after a meal or snack you are hungry again. Is the feeling of hunger what prompts you to seek out food? Or do you simply choose to eat at standard mealtimes or when food is around, regardless of whether you are hungry? I recommend you use a piece of paper or the notepad on your phone to make a list of your eating moments during the day, and note "yes" or "no" to the question of whether you were hungry before eating.

One of the biggest challenges to starting a fasting practice is the fear of being hungry. It might surprise you to learn that you're not always hungry when you reach for food—and perhaps this will give you the confi¬dence to try and skip a meal without fear.

Set clear goals: Why are you interested in fasting in the first place? What exactly do you want to achieve? Be specific. "Lose weight" or "be healthy" are not specific goals. You want to set goals that are clear and easy to measure. I am not a fan of scales, because they can't tell you what portion of your weight is fat and what portion is lean mass. I find that how your clothes fit is a much better gauge of success with fat loss. So take some time to write or think about why you are doing this. Envision your success. You might say: "In six months with intermittent fasting, doing a 24-hour fast two times a week, I will fit into those pants." (You know which pants.) If at three months you are not halfway to your goal, you can adjust.

It also helps to find role models for success. Whom do you know who has done what you want to do? What does their success look like? Decide what you want, envision your success, and go after it.

If you're not sure how to get started, then just start: It's pretty easy to get started. If you are someone who eats three meals a day like clockwork, then start by skipping breakfast tomorrow, and the day after that. If you just ate lunch and feel very full, skip dinner tonight. If you are super motivated right now and want to get started with a 24-hour fast, don't eat again until lunch tomorrow. You really can start now. No time like the present.

How To Practice Intermittent Fasting

When someone first starts fasting, they usually have a few questions: "Exactly how many hours it will take to get into ketosis?" "What level of ketosis should I aim for?" "How long do I have to fast for maximum fat burn¬ing?" These are all reasonable questions, but difficult to answer in a general sense. Many things influence the rate of ketone production; for instance, the amount of liver glycogen you had going into your fast (which is affected by how much carbohydrate you ate prior to fasting). If you typically eat a low-carb or ketogenic diet, then you won't lay down much glycogen at all and you'll enter a ketogenic state more quickly. The amount of exercise you do while you're fasting has an impact as well. This is pretty obvious, though—the more energy you use in the fasted state, the more fat and ketones will be used because those are your main energy sources during a fast. Your size and body composition matters, too, as well as how fit your muscles are and how good they are at using fats, glucose, and ketones.

So the focus on level of ketosis and exact timing to optimize ketone production is a bit misplaced. What's essential is that you keep up a fasting practice and have a varied exercise practice. Do that, and you will get better at producing and using ketones, and better at using fat directly, too. This is what you want.

It's also hard to tell exactly at what time of day your ketones levels will be highest. If you're looking for some marker to decide how long to fast, pay attention to how you feel. Fasting and ketosis increase your sense of well-being. They make you feel good. The caveat is you have to get through the transition from eating all the time and operating solely on a glucose-based metabolism, to eating less often and training your cells to use fat again. That's why I recommend a minimum six-week commitment to any fasting plan you start.

For the rest of this section, I'm going to outline some of the popular intermittent fasting patterns out there, simply because I think it helps to have some models when you're starting out. This section will also include interviews with people who incorporate intermittent fasting into their own lives, so you can see first-hand accounts of how it works. Remember, don't get too caught up in the precise timing or structure of these patterns. The important thing is to begin a fasting practice that is feasible for you and make it a consistent part of your life. There is no perfect schedule except the one that works for you.

The flexibility of intermittent fasting is one of the things that makes it sustainable for the long term. You can fast no matter what type of diet you follow, and you can choose whatever fasting pattern works for you. I consider it a gift to eaters everywhere!

That said, lots of options can be overwhelming, especially if you're used to traditional diets with strict rules and limitations. There's value in having restrictions, especially when you're starting out. So if you want a short list to pick from, here are your top three choices.

- Option 1: A 16:8 time-restricted eating window

Eat within an eight hour window every day. It's probably best to note the time you finish dinner, and count back eight hours from there—that's your starting time. Don't consume any calories the rest of the time. Water, black coffee, and unsweetened tea are okay to have. Keep this pattern on the weekend, too, if you can. Plan morning activities to keep you busy, especially if your family is home eating breakfast. Stick with this fast for six weeks. If you miss a day here and there, keep going. If, after a couple of weeks, the pattern feels easy, or you're just not hungry for your first meal, lengthen your fast by two hours and see how that goes. On the flip side, if at the end of six weeks this daily pattern is not working for you, consider options 2 or 3.

- Option 2: A 24-hour fast

Pick a day that you want to fast. On that day, you will eat dinner only. The night before, make sure to eat a normal dinner at a reasonable hour, and don't snack afterward. Don't stuff yourself at dinner, because it may make your fast harder the next day. Stick to high-fat foods and quality protein for that meal, and avoid anything sugary or starchy. Before you go to sleep, put a sticky note on your bathroom mirror to remind you when you wake up in the morning that you are fasting that day. If you forget, you're liable to eat breakfast and miss your fasting opportunity! Enjoy your fast for the day, have dinner in the evening, and eat normally the rest of the week. Seven days later, do the 24-hour fast again. Practice this for six weeks. If you love it and want to do more, great—choose a second fasting day during the week. Eventually, if you want, you can choose a third. If, on the other hand, you don't like this pattern at all after six weeks, consider options 1 or 3.

- Option 3: The 5:2 fast

Pick two days on which to eat only 25 percent of the amount you normally eat. So if you normally aim for 2000 calories, that'll be 500 calories for your fasting days. That's a very small vegetable salad with some cheese or a little protein, and oil-based dressing. Or, that's half a piece of salmon with a side of green veg¬etables and half an avocado. Aside from that meal, don't eat anything else that day. Eat normally the rest of the week until your second fasting day, and then eat only 25 percent again on that day. For simplicity's sake, it's good to keep the same two days every week, but if you have a social invitation one week that falls on your fasting day, just move your fast to another day. Stick with this for six weeks. You may find that it's easier to go without eating on your fasting days than to eat the small meal (many people do). If so, skip the meal! If after six weeks you really don't like this pattern, try options 1 or 2.

Time-Restricted Eating

If you are new to intermittent fasting, I recommend you start with time-restricted eating. In this pattern, you eat all your food within a specific window of time each day. Most people start out skipping breakfast and eating dinner at a reasonable hour, i.e., a couple of hours before bedtime (no snacking afterward). If you eat lunch at 12 p.m. and dinner before 8 p.m., you've got yourself a 16-hour fast! This is commonly called the "16:8," because you fast for 16 hours (ideally sleeping half the time), and eat for 8 hours. You're permitted snacks during your eating window, though many people find they're not hungry enough to eat more than two meals in 8 hours' time. Your appetite will likely diminish over time, so be attentive to your needs and don't try to cram in meals when you're not hungry.

The "skip breakfast" schedule is a common one, but it's not the only way to practice this fast. If you are someone for whom breakfast is essential, you can still do the 16:8—just shift your eating window to start earlier in the day. For you, a 9 a.m.–5 p.m. eating window may work best. Alternatively, if your business or social life means that dinners usually happen late, then start your fast later in the day so you have time in the evening to accommodate your last meal. You may find that a 2 p.m.–10 p.m. eating window is the right fit for you. Your goal is simply to have 16 hours of fasting time. You muscles will be relying on fats for energy and sparing glucose for the brain. Insulin levels will have been low for 10 hours or more, making fat more avail¬able as an energy source and allowing ketone production to proceed.

With 16 hours of fasting, you'll have achieved a lot of the metabolic changes— ketosis, insulin reduction, growth hormone spike—that you are seeking. It is two-thirds of a day, and it's a great amount of time to be in the fasted state. That said, if you're challenged to meet the 16-hour fasting goal, then simply start with less and work your way up. Soon, you will find that the biggest obstacle to fasting is a psychological one. Start with a 12-hour fast if that's what you feel you can do right now (and remember, eight hours are sleep time), and simply delay your first meal by an hour every few days. I believe you'll be able to work up to a 16-hour fast in no time.

One of the benefits of time-restricted eating is that it may work in synergy with your circadian rhythm. This is the "internal clock" that responds to light and dark and influences physiological signals such as sleepiness, wakefulness, and hunger. There's good evidence that eating during daylight hours is best for our metabolic health, whereas eating at night (when our internal clock wants us to be sleeping) is not so good. If you think about it, for most of human history, eating had to be done during the day because there was no artificial light by which to eat at nighttime. This pattern works with the natural circadian rhythm.

Another benefit of time-restricted eating is that it eliminates the common problem of late-night snacking. When your eating window closes at 8 p.m., there's no peeking in the cabinets for a nibble just before bed. The rules are clear: no eating outside your eating window, which means dinner is the last eating moment of the day. At night, herbal teas are a very good treat.

Lengthening a Daily Fast

Whether you start with a fast of 16 hours or work your way up to it, you may find after a couple of weeks that you can go longer. If you fast in the early part of the day, you'll notice that you're not always hungry when your first mealtime comes around. You may be excited about your progress and feeling empowered, which may give you the motivation to wait another two hours before breaking your fast. After having skipped breakfast every day without trouble, you'll want to challenge yourself to skip lunch some days too—espe¬cially if you were someone who thought you could never manage to skip breakfast even once! Without even realizing, you might make it to dinnertime and discover you haven't eaten since yesterday. This is how people come to dive deeper into the daily fasting pattern, shortening their daily eating window to six, four, or even two hours. The 18:6 or 20:4 are quite popular and relatively easy to maintain, at least during the weekdays. Fat burning is quite high in the 18 to 24 hour period of your fast, so it is worth shooting for that length of time on many or most fasting days. If you don't have a lot of lean body mass (e.g., if you're female and/or you have a high body fat ratio) then you may find more fat-burning success extending your fast to 36 hours.

Some people follow the One Meal A Day (OMAD) pattern, which is akin to a 22- or 23-hour fast every sin¬gle day (23:1), depending on how long you give yourself to eat your one meal. If you're going out to dinner and having appetizers and an entree, for instance, then you may not want to squeeze the whole experience into one hour, so you'll give yourself two hours. Conversely, some people are super strict about their fasting times and stick to a timed eating window every day, at the same time, with no exceptions. If that's your style, then go for it, but don't feel you need to be so strict. It's not going to mess up your ketosis or impede your fat loss if you fast less one day or eat at a different time another day. As mentioned previously, the exact number of hours to achieve a given level of ketosis will vary from person to person and will be influenced by your previous meals, level of exercise or energy spent that day, and other factors.

One of the major benefits of eating once a day is that it is simple and doesn't require you to think about an eating schedule. You get back a lot of time and mental energy that would have otherwise been spent on figuring out what and when to eat. The downside to OMAD is that it lacks variability in energy intake, which can lead to weight plateau. Think about it: if you eat only once a day, you'll probably be eating about the same number of calories day in and day out, and you'll be eating fewer calories than you would if you ate multiple meals per day. This looks a lot like a calorie-restricted diet—the very kind that cause weight plateau. For this reason, one meal a day is a good pattern to stick with for weight maintenance. If you are eating one meal a day and hit a plateau when you still want to be losing weight, go ahead and switch things up. You can add a 36- or 48-hour fast into your week, or a three day fast every other week, for example, and include a couple of days where you eat more than one meal so you can have a much more varied energy intake.

What's important is that you get a command of intermittent fasting and include it in your life in ways that suit you. The precise timing of meals or fasting windows that will lead to "optimal" fat loss matters less than just getting some fasting time in, period. I recommend finding a pattern that fits with your schedule so meals are convenient, and fasting time doesn't disrupt your life. Choose something you will be able to maintain consis¬tently. When needed, make adjustments or vary the schedule to continue to achieve your goals.

Fast a Couple Times Each Week

You don't have to stick to a time-restricted eating window every day in order to practice intermittent fasting. If your work responsibilities mean you'll have to join colleagues for dinner at varying times, or if you have an active social life that includes dining out, then it may be tough for you to keep a daily eating window. Don't worry—you can organize fasts on days of the week when your schedule permits. Part of the beauty of intermittent fasting is its flexibility.

On the popular 5:2 diet, you eat normally five days a week and fast for two days each week. If not eating for an entire day sounds intimidating, keep in mind that you don't have to exclude all meals on a given day. You just have to arrange for a fasting period of a full 24 hours. For example, if one of your fasting days is Thursday, you can eat dinner on Wednesday night, wrapping up by 8 p.m. You fast Thursday morning and afternoon, and plan for dinner to start at around 8 p.m. Thursday night. That way, you'll fast from dinner Wednesday until dinner Thursday, for a total of 24 hours. Do the same for your other fasting day, from dinner to dinner. You'll have fasted 48 hours that week! Eat normally the rest of the week, and repeat the pattern every week.

Pick fasting days that makes sense for your life. You might pick two days that are always hectic at work, because you like being busy while you're fasting. Plan to do some errands or exercise in the evening, and come home properly hungry for your meal those nights. Or maybe you have a day each week that calls out to you as the day you like to rest. This could even be associated with a social or religious practice, such as keeping Sabbath on Saturday, or resting from work on Sunday. You may discover that a fast, or "rest" from eating, is a nice addition to your practice on that day. The important thing is not which days you choose; it's that you choose them, and stick with them week after week.

If you really want to hit the ground running, try a 24-hour fast three days per week. Fast on Monday, Wednesday, and Friday (or whatever schedule works for you). As you get accustomed to the pattern—and your shrinking waist size—you'll find it surprisingly doable. Another riff on this pattern is called alternate-day fasting, and it is as simple as it sounds: eat one day, fast the next. There is a nice rhythm to it. A lot of the benefits we attribute to intermittent fasting come from studies using alternate-day fasting in both animals and humans. It's a good approach from a metabolic standpoint, but it is somewhat impractical because there are an odd number of days every week—which means your fasting days will change every week. It's a lot easier, I think, to pick three fasting days a week and stick with them.

Some versions of full-day fasts allow for a small meal that provides about 25 percent of your normal calorie needs (i.e., about 400 to 600 calories). This is not going to undo all the benefits of the fast, but it can be tricky to consume food on your fasting days. First, it's hard to gauge the number of calories in a meal, and it's very easy to eat more than you think you're eating. It can also be a slippery slope—once you start eating, you may just want to continue, and before you know it, your fasting day has turned into an eating day. But, it is nice to have a backup plan in case the fast is feeling particularly difficult that day. So, take the option to have the small amount of food if you think it will help you get more fasting time overall.

Infrequent Fasts

Fasting on a regular schedule helps you establish a routine and makes fasting a part of your life. Sometimes it's nice to go deeper into the practice every so often. Maybe you want to schedule a three-day or even a five-day fast once a month or every other month to amplify the benefits. Not everyone is going to be able (or excited) to do this, and that's perfectly okay! Even if you don't schedule something of the sort, keep your mind open to possibilities. For example, if you have a week of heavy eating with friends in town or a family gather¬ing, you might be ready to try a few days of fasting the next week. If you do a multi-day fast, you can always consider the option of simply having 25 percent of your normal calories on fasting days.

As I've said before, you really can choose what works for you. If you are like most Westerners, you have spent the majority of your life eating three meals a day, every day, and more when the opportunity presents itself. Any additional time spent fasting is a gift to your body, mind, and soul. If you stick to time-restricted eating for your regular fasting practice and pick just one full day a month for a dedicated fast on top of that, that's a very nice bonus. It all adds up.

Yearly fasts are another option. If you are fasting to lose weight, then a once a year fast is probably not going to help you achieve your long-term goals. That said, a yearly fasting practice can be very beneficial as a meditation or time of reflection, distinct from the practice you maintain of fasting for weight loss. Many reli¬gious and cultural traditions designate particular times of the year for fasting with the goal of slowing down and resting, reflecting, and rejuvenating. In our modern, hectic times, a yearly fast can be a very powerful relaxation tool.

Like a vacation, a yearly fasting practice of even a few days can offer a significant sense of peace and rejuvenation.

Not surprisingly, a common practice on wellness retreats is for participants to fast or eat very lightly. This may be combined with a spiritual or mindfulness practice such as meditation, or a physical one such as yoga. Going on a retreat where fasting is a part of the program is a smart way to familiarize yourself with a meditative fasting practice. These programs provide a structured day and ongoing guidance from retreat leaders so that practitioners are not left on their own. There's a community of people sharing the experience together, many of whom are new to the practice themselves. This sort of environment makes it easy to go along with the new eating patterns and other practices, even if those things would be unfamiliar in your home setting.

Breaking a Fast

People always want to know what they can "eat" on their fast. That's easy: Nothing. Eat nothing! You are fasting. That's the point.

You cannot drink anything with calories (juice, soda, "vitamin water," coconut water, etc.), nor can you drink "diet beverages" without calories (diet soda, diet vitamin water, diet anything). You cannot have gum, suck¬ing candy, breath mints, Tic Tacs, or anything of the sort. If you're following the sort of plan that allows for a small meal (approximately 500 calories) once a day, then you will eat only that meal, and won't have food outside of that.

You must, however, drink a good amount of water. You can have also have unflavored carbonated water. And you can have coffee and tea, unsweetened (including fake sweeteners), and without milk.

How To Take Care Of Yourself With Intermittent Fasting

Fasting for short periods of time is safe and simple for healthy adults. No special preparation or changes to your daily activities are required. You just choose periods of time not to eat, and go about your normal busi¬ness while fasting. Once you start doing research you'll find dozens of websites and videos detailing "secret tips for optimizing your fast," from drinking apple cider vinegar to supplementing with branched chain amino acids (BCAAs) or medium-chain triglyceride (MCT) oil. But there's no need to make this more complicated than it needs to be! While none of these tips are harmful, they're also not necessary— and they can create a lot of extra work and confusion, making fasting seem much more difficult than it really is. The more compli¬cated it is, the less likely you are to stick with it. It's best to keep things simple.

In your research, you might also come across articles obsessing over electrolyte imbalance and scary information about something called "refeeding syndrome." If I were new to fasting and had no background in metabolic science, I would be turned off to the whole thing. But these are not important concerns for healthy adults who practice intermittent fasting and eat an adequate diet otherwise. There are some good practices for taking care of yourself on your fast, which we'll review in this section. For example, drinking broth is a good practice for multi-day fasts. You can take some supplements if you notice they make you feel better. But it's really not essential to do any of that. People all over the world fast all the time without con¬suming special foods or supplements to prepare, and do just fine.

Drink Enough Fluids

If you recall from what I said earlier, fasting depletes glycogen stores, and a lot of water is lost with the glycogen. This accounts for some weight loss and can also result in dehydration if you're not mindful of replenishing your fluids. This is doubly important if you're on a ketogenic diet, because you won't replenish glycogen or its associated water when you eat.

A lot of us are so busy that we don't pay much attention to drinking water throughout the day. Hydration is extremely important on a fast, and you can end up feeling really terrible if you forget to drink enough water on your fasting days. Carbonated water, also called seltzer, club soda, or sparkling water, is a great treat when fasting. It's a little more exciting than regular water, and it's a nice thing to order if you're out at a restaurant and don't want to eat or drink.

In addition to water and carbonated water, herbal tea is a great option when fasting. Herbal tea is made from the dried leaves of flowers and herbs, and doesn't have caffeine. It is hydrating, and you can drink as much as you like! Examples are chamomile, rooibos, lavender, mint, and dandelion root. Be sure to read the ingredient list and avoid teas that include ground ingredients like cacao that contain calories, or those that include sweeteners. You can also drink caffeinated tea, but of course, you will feel the effects of the caffeine. Black tea, green tea, oolong, and fermented teas are all good to have, but, like coffee, you will have a toler¬ance limit for the caffeine and won't want to drink too much of it, or drink it at night. That's where the herbal teas come in handy!

Some people incorporate bone broth, such as chicken or beef broth, into their fasting regimen, especially if they are doing multi-day fasts and find it challenging to go without food entirely during that time. For very few calories (100 to 200 per bowl), they can drink some broth and feel rejuvenated. It is hydrating (good when you're fasting), provides minerals and electrolytes (it's good to salt your broth), and provides some amino acids as well. The smell and taste of the broth can relieve hunger. Of course, because broth does deliver nutrients to the body, it will trigger nutrient sensors that tell the body you are no longer fasting. A small rise in insulin should occur. This is a small effect relative to eating a meal, so it's not a total loss—and many people find that they are able to fast longer if they include broth in their fasting days, so the trade-off works out in the end. However, it doesn't make sense to have broth for fasts of a day or less since most people can go that long without eating and feel just fine—and the whole point of a fasting practice is to actually fast during your fasting time! Either way, broth is good to consume during your eating window to get the benefits of hydration and a dose of minerals.

Consume Sodium, Potassium, and Magnesium Regularly

Electrolytes are minerals that perform essential functions in the body, such as moving nutrients into and out of cells, supporting nerve impulses, and supporting muscle contractions, including those of the heart muscle. The function of these minerals is very well regulated in a healthy person. Sodium, potassium, and magnesium are all electrolytes. Their concentration depends a lot on the amount of water in the body, and therefore dehydration (or overhydration) can cause an imbalance of electrolytes.

You hear a lot about sodium in connection with fasting and ketogenic dieting because your kidneys excrete more sodium while you're fasting, and levels of potassium and magnesium can be affected too. The best way to ensure you have enough sodium, potassium, and magnesium is to consume these minerals in your diet. Contrary to conventional wisdom, do not be afraid of salt! There is good evidence to suggest that lim¬iting sodium to about 2000 mg per day is not ideal and can be harmful. Sodium needs for someone who is fasting, or on a ketogenic diet, are much higher, between 3000 to 5000 mg per day. I generally discourage calculating nutrient intakes unless you are managing a health problem that requires nutrient monitoring (e.g., diabetes, kidney disease) or are using diet to enhance athletic performance and seeking a narrow range of intake. For the majority of us just trying to have a healthy diet and avoid weight gain, it's quite cumbersome to track how much sodium we consume every day! It's simplest to focus on adding salt to your diet. Put salt on your food and use it liberally when cooking. If you drink broth, salt your broth. If you eat avocados, cucumber slices, or tomato slices on their own, sprinkle salt on them! It's delicious, and will help you main¬tain a good sodium level.

Magnesium and potassium are found in varying amounts in nearly all types of whole foods. Focus your diet on vegetables, meat and fish, high-quality dairy, nuts, and some fruits. Nuts like almonds and cashews are rich in magnesium, as are avocados, green vegetables, salmon and other fish, and dairy products. Potassium is found in dark green leafy vegetables, dairy products, meat and fish, legumes like lentils and beans, winter squash, sweet potatoes, some nuts and seeds, and dried fruit.

Most adults in the United States consume less magnesium and less potassium than is recommended. Magnesium deficiency can cause fatigue, weakness, and muscle cramps. If you notice these symptoms, you can take a magnesium supplement of up to 400 mg per day. Potassium deficiency can cause similar symp¬toms of muscle cramps and twitching, as well as irregular heart rate. Potassium supplements are not very common, as taking too much can be dangerous. It's best to eat a diet rich in the foods mentioned.

If you're only fasting for periods of a day or less and eating mineral-rich foods on your eating days, then it's not likely you will have a problem with electrolytes. If you are fasting in combination with a ketogenic diet, then you may have to pay closer attention and look out for symptoms of electrolyte imbalance.

Break Your Fast with Something Small

It's a good idea to eat a small meal or snack to break your fast, and see whether you have the appetite for a full meal. You don't have to eat any special foods, but you simply may not have room for much right away. If you're fasting for a day or less, there's no harm to breaking your fast with a typical meal if that's what works in your schedule—you just may notice that you can't finish it, and choose to put the rest away for later. If you're fasting for a couple of days, then it's more important to go slowly when you start to eat again. Have something light that's not too hard on the digestive tract. A common tradition for breaking the fast of Ramadan is to eat one date, the sugary fruit of the date palm that you may know better in its dried version. This small dose of sugar gets digestive juices flowing and prepares the body to receive more food. I am not exactly a fan of sugary things, so I prefer to have just a few bites of a meal and wait a while until I've grown an appetite for the rest. You might want to break your fast with a small cup of broth-based soup (cream-based is tougher on the digestive tract), a small green salad, or something else that you know agrees with you. I recommend avoiding fried foods, very acidic foods (like tomato sauce or orange juice), large amounts of sugar or flour (e.g., cake, cookies, pasta), and dairy products, as these tend to cause bloating and upset stomach if eaten after a period of fasting.

Cut Down on Your Alcohol Consumption

If you do drink alcohol, give some thought to how and whether you want to modify your drinking habits to accommodate your new fasting habit. (If you're not a drinker, good for you! That's one less thing to tackle.) I notice that folks who drink seem to be in two camps when it comes to modifying their drinking patterns to start an intermittent fasting practice. On the one hand, there are those who want to cut out drinking entirely as part of their new diet habits. They'll have it easier when they start fasting, and depending on the amount they drink, will likely lose more weight without the alcohol. The other group doesn't want to cut out drinking, but may cut down in amount or frequency. They'll have to do a bit more scheduling work, because alcohol can make fasting a bit trickier. Know that alcohol will affect your appetite in unpredictable ways, both on the day you're drinking, and the day after. So if you drink alcohol at night and expect to fast the next day, you may be in for an unpleasant fast. Alcohol is dehydrating, and fasting is too, so you'll need even more fluid on your fast. If drinking alcohol makes you to want to binge on starchy foods, well, you may just be playing with fire there. These are just considerations for you. Use common sense about how drinking will affect your fasting practice, and make adjustments that help you achieve the goals that matter to you. Alcohol is by no means "banned." If you're someone who is disciplined with drinking and your alcohol consumption consists of one glass of wine or a cocktail at dinner, you'll be able to gauge how the drink affects your fast and figure out the best way to work around it. If you drink more heavily, then you may want to consider cutting down.

Take Time to Adjust

Fasting increases adrenaline levels, readying the body for action. That's because fasting, like exercise, is a mild form of stress that results in some positive changes in the body. While fasting, noradrenaline helps the body focus strength and resources on getting through the "challenge"—that is, it gives you energy and mental focus to go out and find food. Remember, the body's hormonal system doesn't know we have gro¬cery stores now; it thinks we still have to go out and hunt animals for food! So adrenaline increases your heart and metabolic rates, and releases stored glucose and fat into the bloodstream to provide energy for the hunt. This is, of course, very good for weight loss, but it's not always good for sleeping. If, during your fasting window, you find that you're jittery, have trouble falling asleep, or wake up abruptly in the middle of the night, it's likely that adrenaline is the culprit. Take steps to minimize the impact of this hormone on your schedule. You may want to quit drinking caffeine for a while, and practice sleep meditation or take a nightly bath to put you in a calm mood before bed. Take advantage of the extra energy and focus to be more productive and tackle tasks that have been on your to-do list for a while, even if that means knock¬ing them out at odd hours of the night. And remember—adrenaline is keeping your metabolic rate high, and your body burning through more fat. Hopefully that's motivation enough to make it through the energy highs if they're bothersome to you.

Don't Start Fasting in Periods of High Stress

You're probably familiar with the hormone cortisol. Cortisol, like adrenaline, is produced in the body as a response to stress and is meant to help focus the body's faculties on overcoming the stress and returning to normal. The relevant difference is that cortisol levels can remain high over a long period of time if the body is under chronic stress. One of cortisol's main functions is to trigger the release of glucose into the blood. Insulin levels rise in response. In a momentarily stressful situation, this system would provide the body with energy needed to fight or flee whatever stressor it faced. But persistently elevated cortisol levels can keep blood sugar and insulin levels persistently high and lead to weight gain and insulin resistance. If you are in a period of high stress in your life—whether because of a job change, relationship troubles, an illness, or other difficult time— then it's probably not the best time to start your fast. If you're eager to get started anyway, then keep to the time-restricted eating approach (fast for 16 hours and eat within an 8-hour window every day) and avoid longer fasts until the stress has subsided.

Exercise on Empty

I get asked all the time if it's okay to work out "on an empty stomach." The answer is yes! It is safe and per¬fectly normal for the average person to do some exercise without having had any food. In general, a healthy adult will not have adverse reactions to exercising on an empty stomach. If you're seeking weight loss, then working out without eating will help you burn through fat more quickly—even more so if you've already done an overnight fast. Plus, as we discussed above, adrenaline levels are higher when you fast, so you'll likely have more energy to commit to your exercise routine if you choose to exercise fasted.

That said, if you are someone who has a history of feeling weak, faint, or dizzy after exercise on an empty stomach, and you know that it's not the right thing for you, then don't do it. Pay attention to your body, and don't do something that makes you feel bad. If fasted workouts don't suit you, it's certainly wise to arrange an exercise schedule that fits with your fasting schedule in a way that allows you to feel good while doing both. One of the great things about fasting, as I've said before, is you can pretty much arrange it how you like. Just pick a time to fast that doesn't conflict with the training you want to do.

For the rest of us, exercising on empty is a nice hack that can speed fat loss. I would hate for you to miss out on it because you've been taught that you'll become dangerously hypoglycemic if you don't have a pre-workout, carb-based snack. Consider this: many adults all over the world perform some type of manual labor in the course of their day just to make a living, get around, or provide sustenance for their families. Many communities in Africa, Asia, and South America practice subsistence farming and walk long distances to get basic necessities like water and cooking fuel. And many of them do this without obsessing over what to eat before their "workout." The human body is not as fragile as you may think.

How To Eat When It's Time To Eat

Intermittent fasting is only half the fun. The other half is intermittent eating! And when you eat, you must eat well. On your eating days, eat to satisfaction! I often see people get so excited about their progress and the fact that they're able to go a whole day without eating that they think to themselves, "Oh, I'll just go light on this meal," and the next meal, and the next. Or they avoid fat when they eat because it's calorie dense and they think that keeping calories low all the time will speed their weight loss. Or they find some other strategy that amounts to alternating bouts of fasting with bouts of calorie-restricted eating. This is a mistake! This approach will result in the dreaded slowdown of metabolism that causes weight plateau and regain. Instead, focus on getting a wide variation in energy intake—from no energy one day while you're fasting, to lots of energy the next day while you're eating.

I'm not going to dive into a big explanation of why you should eat mostly whole, unprocessed foods. Collectively, we are very aware that the average American diet based on processed foods and lots of sugar is making us fat and sick. If you've read this far into a book about how to lose weight and improve your health, then you're already highly motivated to jump off that bandwagon. It's especially important to eat a robustly nutritious diet when you practice intermittent fasting because you have to get all your nourishment in a shorter window of time. To do this, eat what you want, as long as what you're eating has been grown on trees, from the ground, or in the seabed, or was once a living animal, and hasn't been altered much on its way to your plate. Whatever you're eating, put salt on it. Most people would benefit from eating more fat and fewer carbs. Don't overdo the protein. Avoid processed and packaged foods at all costs. And don't eat anything cooked in "vegetable oil."

Eat a Good Amount of Fat

Fat is satiating, so you stay full longer after a meal with fat than one without it. Fat doesn't increase insulin levels, so it won't contribute to insulin resistance the ways carbs will. If you've struggled with weight loss on a low-fat diet in the past, or you have poor discipline when it comes to carbohydrates, then focus on getting more fat and pushing some of the carbs off your plate. There are different types of fats, and optimal health is achieved by eating a variety of fats. Here's a quick review:

Monounsaturated fats are found in high amounts in avocados and olives and their oils, and most nuts and seeds. These fats are a cornerstone of the Mediterranean diet and are linked to lower risk of heart disease. As a rule of thumb, it's good to eat more monounsaturated fat.

Saturated fats are found in fatty portions of foods from land animals, such as the skin of a chicken, the marbling of a steak, or the extra fat in bacon or pork belly. Butter and dairy products are also high in satu¬rated fat. The only plant foods rich in saturated fat are coconut and palm oils. Saturated fat has long been demonized because it was believed to be a major cause of heart disease, but that theory has not proved true. There is no reason to avoid saturated fat. However, many people fail to consume other types of fat and get most of their fat in the form of saturated fat, which isn't ideal. It's important to vary your fat intake. So if you tell me you don't like fish or avocado and just want to get all your fat from bacon and steak, I'll tell you to be a little more open minded. Try some new things!

Polyunsaturated fats are found in plant foods and fish, and there are two types that are important to differ¬entiate: omega-3 fats, which most people need to consume more of, and omega-6 fats, which practically everyone needs to consume less of. The balance of omega-3 and omega-6 fats is extremely important for overall health, and excess omega-6 fats contribute to inflammation and diseases associated with it, includ¬ing obesity, diabetes, and cardiovascular disease.

Incorporating Fat into Your Diet

I recommend cooking everything in olive oil unless you're looking for a specific flavor from butter, animal fat, or coconut oil. There's a misguided belief that olive oil should only be used for cold preparations because it doesn't have a high smoke point, but it's perfectly okay to use olive oil for baking, roasting, or sautéing foods. I wouldn't use olive oil for frying, but then again, I wouldn't recommend frying your food. Use olive oil for salad dressings, as well. Drizzle olive oil on top of any finished meal that's light on fat.

Eat avocados: Avocados are a uniquely high-fat, nutrient-rich fruit, and I recommend you make them a regular part of your diet. If you live in a part of the world where avocados are not easy to get in the regular supermarket, visit a Latin American grocery store in your vicinity. There, you will find avocados, most likely ripe and reasonably priced. You can buy a few at a time and leave them in the fridge if they are close to ripe or out on the counter for a couple of days if they're not. Eat avocados sliced on the side of your meal, or make avocado mash or guacamole regularly. Use avocados in sauces or dressings to thicken them. If you're really not a fan of avocados, include avocado oil in your diet. Both avocados and olives (as well as their oils) are high in monounsaturated fat that most people would benefit from eating more of.

Use liberal amounts of olive, avocado, and coconut oil or butter in your cooking. Fat transfers heat from the pan to the food, allowing for well-rounded cooking. Fat also carries flavor and adds moisture to a dish—you will notice a significant difference in flavor when you use a good amount of oil to sauté leafy greens, for instance, rather than just enough oil to coat the bottom of the pan. Don't be afraid to use a lot of fat when cooking! This is the secret to flavor in restaurant dishes, because chefs are not afraid of fat at all. Don't just leave a piece of meat or a portion of vegetables naked on your plate. Finish dishes with fat-rich sauces or dressings like tahini or cream sauce, or oil-based condiments like pesto or chimichurri.

There are other simple ways to get more fat in your diet. If you eat dairy products like yogurt and cheese, always choose the full-fat version. Always eat whole eggs rather than just egg whites. Swap out grain flours, such as wheat, for nut flours, such as almond, in baking recipes. Include a handful of nuts before or after a meal that doesn't contain a lot of fat. Use full-fat, pure coconut milk instead of dairy milk or processed nut or grain milks (e.g., almond, oat) in smoothies, curries, or any desserts you make.

Eat Protein in Moderation

More is not necessarily better when it comes to protein. The average person in the United States consumes more protein than needed to meet their needs. We are accustomed to a large piece of meat on our plate—usually with a double serving of starch and a stingy portion of vegetables. This is a distorted view of what a meal should be. Aim for a little less meat, way less starch, and more green vegetables (unless you're on a ketogenic diet, which we'll discuss below).

Lean toward fattier cuts of meats so you can achieve higher fat intake. Eat the dark meat and the skin of the chicken rather than just a breast—and no skinless breasts, please! Select marbled cuts of beef such as rib eye over lean cuts like sirloin, and talk to the butcher to get more familiar with the fat content of the cuts available at your grocer. Look for ground beef with an 80/20 ratio of lean meat to fat rather than a 90/10 ratio. Opt for lamb instead of beef when you can find it. Choose fatty fish like salmon and mackerel over lean fish like sole/flounder, tilapia, or cod, and eat the skin of the fish too. Enjoy bacon and pork belly instead of leaner cuts like pork tenderloin or pork chop. If you like organ meats like heart, liver, and other innards, eat those for their high fat and/or high mineral content. Broth made from the bones of beef, chicken, or other animal is a good source of the minerals that are important during fasting, and also provides some protein and a small amount of fat.

Eggs and dairy products also provide some protein, as do nuts and seeds. Legumes such as lentils, black beans, or chickpeas are good vegan protein sources.

Eat Non-Starchy Vegetables

Since you're fasting to lower insulin levels and allow fat burning to happen, it's not a great idea to eat a lot of carb-heavy foods like bread, potatoes, rice, sweet potatoes, or other starches, or to consume sugary foods like desserts or sweetened beverages (including sugar in your tea or coffee). That will just result in high blood sugar, followed by high insulin levels and renewed hunger when blood sugar falls back down. You'll eat again—and mostly carbs—soon after you've digested your meal, triggering another round of high insulin and quickly renewed hunger. This is the cycle that leads to insulin resistance and weight gain in the first place!

It's better to eat fewer carbs, and more nutritious ones, which you can do by focusing on non-starchy veg¬etables along with small amounts of starches and fruit (though, if you're eating a ketogenic diet, you won't consume starch or fruit at all). These foods contribute fiber, water, and vitamins and minerals to your diet, all essential to supporting weight loss and maintaining good health.

Eat lots of leafy greens like spinach, arugula, salad greens, mustard greens, bok choy, and kale. Eat other brassicas like broccoli, Brussels sprouts, cabbage, and cauliflower. Think of cucumber slices or blanched asparagus spears instead of chips or bread when you need something to dip into, say, guacamole or hummus. Wild mushrooms are an excellent addition to most people's diets, as they are low in calories and high in lots of micronutrients, plus they're delicious and have a "meaty" or umami flavor when cooked. Sea vegetables like algae are highly nutritious and often forgotten about in our culture. If you're not familiar, try a seaweed salad the next time you're at a restaurant that serves one, as you may find you like it! You can also add spirulina, a powdered form of seaweed, to smoothies. Use alliums like garlic and onion; roots like gin¬ger, turmeric, and horseradish; and herbs like basil, cilantro, thyme and rosemary in your cooking, as these plant foods have great medicinal properties and add layers of flavor to your food.

Foods To Avoid

In general, don't eat any food that your great-great-grandmother wouldn't recognize as food. Another rule of thumb is to make sure the food hasn't been changed much from its original form, and that the original is recognizable in the final product. Take apple juice as an example. Looking at a glass of apple juice, can you tell it came from an apple? Not really, so I wouldn't consume it. What about canned whole tomatoes? They look pretty much like raw tomatoes, only they're cooked. They pass the test. An exception to this rule is olive and coconut oils, which don't look like olives or coconuts at all! These foods are good to eat, and you should look for the word "virgin" on the label to make sure they're not processed more than necessary.

Avoid Processed Foods

I don't eat or recommend that others eat processed foods—yes, technically, fermented vegetables and cured meats are processed foods because of the methods used to transform them from their raw, natural states into their final form, but that's not what I'm talking about here. When I say processed foods, I mean things in a box or package with a Nutrition Facts panel on them. Cereal, crackers, microwavable mac and cheese, frozen burritos, and jarred sauces made thick with xanthan gum are examples of the types of foods I am talking about. For simplicity's sake, I'll refer to these types of processed foods as "junk food."

I'll give a special mention here to "bars." Do not eat "bars." Food bars, energy bars, breakfast bars, meal replacement bars, whatever-you-want-to-call-them-bars—avoid these at all costs. Bars are just amalgama¬tions of some sugar (agave nectar, date paste, evaporated cane juice, or sugar by some other fancy name) smushed together with some nuts or seeds and sprinkled with protein powder. They honestly remind me of the concentrated food pellets used to fatten up mice in the biochemistry lab I worked in after college. You, a human being, should eat real food. Please.

Your appetite for having real, nourishing food over junk food is improved when you fast. Once you go half a day or more without eating, when the time comes, you are ready for something wholesome. That said, if you eat a junk food diet despite this, intermittent fasting will probably help mitigate the effects of your poor food choices on your health. So if you are unable or unwilling to cut out these foods, then at a minimum, you should incorporate an intermittent fasting practice into your life.

Avoid Seed Oils

Seed oils are oils extracted from the seed of any plant as opposed to its fruit. Earlier, I recommended using olive, avocado, or coconut. These oils are produced from the fruit of the tree and produce healthy oils with a beneficial nutrient profile. In contrast, seed oils are produced from plant seeds such as soybeans, cot¬tonseed, or corn kernels, and are much too high in inflammatory omega-6 fats. "Vegetable oil" is usually a mixture of these and is an equally bad choice. Moreover, these oils are industrially produced (i.e., you can't make them in your home kitchen), and that extra processing does not work in our favor when it comes to dietary health. Finally, these oils are extremely cheap and don't spoil very easily—making them an excellent choice for use in prepared and processed food products that are optimized for cheap production and long shelf-life.

You probably consume a lot of seed oils if you often eat out at restaurants or eat packaged foods. It's best to eliminate unnecessary sources of seed oils from your diet. When eating out, ask about the types of oils they use in the kitchen, and steer toward those that use olive oil, butter, or animal fats. If you have bottles of vegetable oil in your home, toss them now.

Avoid Alcohol

Alcohol obviously isn't a category of food. I've included it here because alcohol contains calories, which means it provides energy and can promote weight gain just like other calorie-containing ingestible. Many people believe that the calories in alcoholic beverages come solely from sweeteners and juice-based mixers added to them. That's not true. Alcohol provides 7 cal per gram all on its own. Any juice, sugar, or syrup added to the drink will tack on additional calories in the form of carbohydrates. Drinks made with egg white will also have protein calories, while those made with cream will additional have fat calories.

The internet would have you believe that certain spirit alcohols, such as vodka or gin, are calorie-free or "not as fattening" as other spirits—or, my personal favorite, that vodka and other colorless spirits have fewer carbs than whiskey, rum, and other amber-colored ones. Let's set the record straight once and for all: distilled spirits do not contain carbohydrates in any amount whatsoever. Zero. No carbs. No fat or protein, either. That's because spirits are produced in a process called distillation, in which a fermented mash of carbohydrate is heated so that the liquid (ethanol) boils and becomes a gas, travels through a tube, cools, transforms back into a liquid and settles into a new container. The mash containing all the carbohydrate is left behind in the old container. You might remember this process from high school chemistry class where you separated salt or another dissolved solid from the liquid in which it was dissolved. It seemed like magic at the time, but now it's just booze (which some might say is magic, too).

Wine and beer are different from distilled spirits in that they do contain some residual carbohydrate from their respective starting products (grapes in the case of wine, and grains in the case of beer). That's because wine and beer are mechanically separated (e.g., filtered) from their starting products and do not go through a distillation process. Below is a chart of average calorie counts and carbohydrate content for common alcoholic beverages.

CHAPTER 7

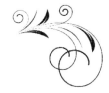

THE KETOGENIC DIET AND FASTING

It's no secret that I'm a fan of both the lower-than-average and very-low-carb/ketogenic approaches. I think the very-low-carb approach brings tremendous benefits to many people, and it's gotten a bad rap for far too long. It might be fun to try if you're already an experienced faster.

That said, don't feel you have to go keto if it really doesn't appeal to you. Some people have dietary prefer¬ences that make keto unfeasible (vegans, for example, would have a very hard time meeting their nutrient needs on a ketogenic diet). But let's be very clear: there is no "kind of" keto or "halfway" keto. You're either on a ketogenic diet or you're not. If you're not, then you're on a low-carb diet, and you'll likely have better weight loss results than anyone on a moderate- or high-carb diet. If you're going keto, then there are some points to review.

What a Ketogenic Diet Is Not

I generally like to focus on what a dietary strategy is and how it works to promote weight loss and pre¬vent disease. I avoid harping on what you can't eat or defining a diet by explaining how it's different than something else. But after countless conversations with individuals who believe they are on a ketogenic diet when they are not, and after reading numerous articles on "how to go keto!" that don't quite capture it, I've decided to take a different approach. The following dietary strategies are not equivalent to a ketogenic diet.

Low-carb is not necessarily keto: On a low-carb diet, you'll avoid foods that we consider starchy or sugary. You won't eat sweets like desserts, pastries, muffins, cookies, candy, or chocolate, or any dried fruits like dried mango, raisins, or others. You won't consume sugary beverages like soda, juice, sweetened tea or coffee, cold-pressed juices, or electrolyte replacement drinks such as Gatorade. You won't eat foods made with grain flour, such as breads, pasta, crackers, or any whole grain foods, including rice, quinoa, couscous, farro, etc. You may also eliminate potatoes and other starchy vegetables including sweet potatoes, winter squash, and corn. You will eat lots of non-starchy vegetables—as much as you want! However, you will not eat unlimited non-starchy vegetables if you're following a ketogenic diet.

High fat is not necessarily keto: Eating lots of fat while also eating lots of carbs is not only not keto, it's terrible for your health. Adding MCT oil to your normal diet does not make you "a keto warrior." Just upping your fat intake—even artificially increasing your blood ketone levels—does not mean you're ketogenic. The genesis part of the word "ketogenic" implies that your body is generating the ketones from your body fat.

High protein is definitely not keto: It's hard to believe that this is still a point of confusion, but it is. A ketogenic diet is one in which your protein intake is low to moderate. It's not a meat-based diet. To do keto properly, you will need to eat smaller portions of meat and focus on fattier cuts—no lean proteins, no egg whites, no skinless chicken breasts.

Cleaning up your diet by eliminating sugary, processed foods is far from keto. You have to make much more dramatic changes than that. Additionally, eating lots of keto junk foods like fat bombs and "keto cake" may technically fit into a ketogenic diet, but I don't recommend it! Aim to eat real food. If it can't be made deli¬cious without a synthetic sweetener like erythritol, it's probably not worth eating.

What Is a Ketogenic Diet?

A ketogenic diet is any diet in which the body is producing ketones at a level high enough to contribute meaningfully to the body's energy needs. This really only happens when your carb intake is exceptionally low, protein intake is low to moderate, and fat intake is extremely high. (Of course, ketones also contribute significantly to energy needs during fasting, but fasting isn't considered a diet so much as it is a break from your diet.) On a ketogenic diet, your macronutrient ratios will be somewhere in the realm of 80 percent calories from fat, 15 percent from protein, and 5 percent from carbs. Another way of approaching the diet is to limit net carbs (total carbs minus fiber) to roughly 20 to 25 grams per day, eat 1 gram of protein per kilogram of body weight, and take the rest of your energy as fat.

The two biggest mistakes I see people make when attempting a ketogenic diet are eating too many veg¬etables and not eating enough fat. What many people seem to misunderstand is that you can't eat all the vegetables you want on a ketogenic diet! You can only have vegetables in very small amounts. This goes counter to everything we think we know about how to eat healthy and lose weight, so most people keep eating lots of vegetables, and they never achieve a ketogenic state!

Vegetables have carbs. Yes—kale, broccoli, and cucumbers all have carbs. Overall, the amount is very small. But you are only permitted a tiny allotment of carbs when you're on a ketogenic diet, so, you can't eat very many vegetables and stay in ketosis. Sure, if you're a keto-adapted athlete, a large man with a lot of lean body mass and a fast metabolism, or you're someone who's been properly intermittent fasting and ketogenic dieting for years, then you can probably get away with eating more vegetables and stay in ketosis or quickly bounce back without much trouble. But I'm guessing if you're reading this book, then you're not one of those super keto-adapted people, so you would have to limit your vegetable intake if you wanted to follow a ketogenic diet.

You also can't eat a lot of protein. Don't have 10-ounce steaks or four chicken thighs at every meal. Protein interferes with ketosis.

So what is left to eat? Fat. Not fat and lots of other stuff that we think of as diet foods, like chicken breast and extra-large kale salads. Just fat. This is hard to comprehend, because we don't eat anything that's pure fat. We don't eat sticks of butter, or spoonfuls of olive oil, or a nice cup of lard. So we really have a hard time wrapping our heads around this concept of a ketogenic diet. But it's quite doable if you are open-minded enough to try it.

Breaking Your Fast

Some of my favorite eating moments happen when I'm fasting, and I wouldn't be doing a complete job if I didn't share some of my favorite meals with you. Breaking my fast is something of an occasion, and I par¬ticipate more fully in the experience of eating. I don't gorge or get greedy when I eat. I just appreciate food more.

Since there are no specific food restrictions with fasting, I'm going to focus on the other major challenge many of us have to eating well: time. I'll walk you through how to prepare dozens of basic meals made from whole foods that are delicious and a lot less labor intensive than you might think. The focus will be on tech¬nique, which is the basis of all good cooking. If you master a few techniques—roasting vegetables, roasting meats, making emulsions or sauces, making stock—then a world of great meals will be open to you.

More than half of recipes that follow are for meals I typically eat, and they are not hard to make. The rest are more complex, for the adventurous among you! I am the first to confess that I am super lazy in the kitchen most of the time. Don't get me wrong—I love to cook when the mood is right. If it's a special occasion that calls for a big meal, like Thanksgiving or a visit from friends who live abroad, then I'll happily spend a few days preparing for the big feast and all day cooking it. If I've recently learned a new technique, like pickling vegetables, I will come home with 17 pounds of produce and enlist the help of friends to turn them into mouth-puckering delights in 32 mason jars that take up two shelves of my fridge for an entire year. In other words, I can really geek out on cooking and food prep when I want to.

However, I am not up for complicated, time-consuming cooking on any given night—especially when my eating window is about to close in one hour. It is very stressful to get home from work and realize you need to eat ASAP, and then set about creating a delicious meal from scratch. It's best to think ahead. So, here are the five cooking rules that get me through life without ever having to order take-out:

1.Whenever you cook, make enough for at least three meals, if not more. Freeze what you can't eat soon. If you've ever made a soup, stew, or casserole (or even a pie, cake, or loaf of bread), you're inherently famil¬iar with the concept of "batch cooking." You invest the time to make a pot of soup just once and know it'll feed you four or five times that week. You don't make one serving of soup from scratch each night for dinner. That would be a waste of time and energy.

Other foods can be batch cooked, too. I often roast a whole chicken, sear off two or three steaks at a time, make an egg frittata in a single pan that can last all week, and sauté three bunches of kale at once. The time saved is significant. For instance, just to prepare the kale, I use four kitchen tools: a cutting board and knife to chop the garlic, and a sauté pan and tongs to cook the kale; these all have to be washed after use, which can be one time if you batch cook, but five or six times if you cook one serving at a time.

The batch cooking method works very well for garnishes and condiments that can hold for months, such as preserved lemons, pickled onions, and pesto (freeze it). When your meal calls for a kick, you'll have a few flavor enhancers to choose from!

2.Use the scraps or leftovers of one meal for another: Our grandmothers didn't throw away chicken carcasses, and neither should we! Instead, we should use them to make a tasty broth for our next soup. Store them in a sturdy zip-top plastic bag in the freezer until you get a few, and spend one day making a few quarts of broth to pull out as needed. You can do the same with lobster bodies and shrimp peels for a seafood broth, and the unwanted ends of vegetables for a vege¬table broth.

When you fry bacon or other fatty meat, collect and strain the fat from the pan and store it in a glass jar in the fridge. You can use the fat when a dish would benefit from a meatier flavor than olive or coconut oil can offer (I like to put bacon fat in a bean casserole, for instance). Be sure to label the jars with a "P" for pork, "L" for lamb, and so on, or you'll go crazy trying to sort them out.

And when you get to that moment there are only two bites of a meal left, stop eating. Put the two bites back in their container in the fridge. You may want to make an omelet the next day, and that small amount of leftovers might just be a nice addition. Or you might end up throwing them out. It's okay.

3.Master the preparation of seven to ten meals: It should be obvious that if you make a meal more than a dozen times, you'll get pretty good at it after a while and it will be easier than it was in the beginning. I find that many home cooks are sometimes too ambitious with their meal prep, trying new dishes on a weeknight from recipes they find on the web. This introduces the challenge of novelty into their food prep and could lead to more time spent, and more stress, than they'd planned for. Unless you are a seasoned cook and really love being in the kitchen, I strongly encourage you to keep it simple. Find a handful of meals that you like, and learn to make them well. Experiment with new dishes when you have lots of time to spare, and keep some leftovers on hand just in case.

4.Simplify recipes that seem too complicated: I rarely follow recipes because they overwhelm me. They tend to include small amounts of lots of different things, and then I have to go buy those things, use them once, and let them go bad in the fridge later that week. Plus, I get tired of measuring and chopping all those different ingredients. I prefer to keep it simple. If a recipe looks good but complicated, my first move is to see which ingredients can be spared. If there's a sauce for the meat, but I can make one with jus and a pad of butter in the same pan, I will probably do that instead. If a recipe calls for parsley and cilantro, I may skip the parsley because it is more neutral in flavor and I probably won't miss it. And no way am I making two starches! There's a recipe I love with tofu, broc¬coli, sweet potatoes, brown rice, and a tahini sauce; I have never once made the rice, as sweet potatoes are quite enough for me. You get the idea. Look for the low-hanging fruit, the thing that won't be missed, and skip it.

5.Buy fresh foods that can be eaten straight from the package: I dislike and strongly discourage what we call "snack" foods. The vast majority of them are shelf-stable, highly processed foods like breakfast cereal, chips, and "energy bars" made of sugar, flour, and hydroge¬nated oils that jeopardize your health. I tell clients to avoid them, period.

But in the sense that snacks are simply foods that don't require any work to prepare, well, there are many that I love. Think fresh, whole foods that would spoil if removed from their package or the refrigerator, but, when stored properly, provide convenient nutrition. Olives, apples, cheese, Persian cucumbers, almonds, unsweetened real yogurt, flaxseed crackers, smoked fish...the list goes on. What's great about many of these is they don't spoil quickly, so you can easily keep them on hand for when they're needed.

Recipes

Whole Roast Chicken

When making a roast chicken, always think about prep for other meals. If there's enough meat left on the carcass, pick it over and pull the bits of meat and skin off. Those small pieces and some of the breast meat can be turned into Chicken Salad with Mayo or Cobb Salad. Put the carcass away in a plastic bag in the freezer. When you have enough carcasses, you'll make a Chicken Broth.

1.Take the chicken out of the fridge and remove entirely from its packaging. Rinse the bird only if you notice any off smells or blood on its skin, and pat it dry with paper towels. Sprinkle salt all over the bird, and place it breast side down on a dish. Let come to room temperature on the counter for about 1 hour, depending on the size of the bird. Halfway through, pat the skin dry all around and flip the bird over so that it's breast side up, and preheat the oven to 450°F. Pat it dry again before you put it in the oven.

2.Place the bird on a baking sheet and cook it alone, with nothing else in the oven. The high temperature may produce a lot of smoke, but it'll be worth it for the delicious crispy skin it creates.

3.Check the temperature of the bird at 35 minutes, and remove when it has an internal temperature of about 155°F, after 45 minutes to an hour. Let the bird rest on the counter for at least 20 minutes; it will keep cooking, and the internal temperature will rise to about 165°F. When it's ready, remove the legs, breast, and wings, and reserve any liquid that's collected in the pan. Eat what you want, and put the other pieces, covered with the excess liquid, away in a glass container for a meal another day.

Asian Variation: Before placing the bird in the oven, place once slice of ginger and one garlic clove between each of the leg joints and wing joints. Sprinkle the outside of the bird with 2 tablespoons of soy sauce and the juice of two lemons. Place the lemon rinds inside the cavity, along with another clove of garlic. Cook as directed.

French Dijon Variation: Place two halved lemons and 4 springs of thyme inside the cavity of the bird before cooking. When the chicken is cooked and resting, make the sauce: To a medium skillet over a high flame, add 2 thinly sliced shallots, ¾ cup dry white wine, and ¾ cup of chicken juices from the roasting pan. Reduce the mixture by half, 2 to 3 minutes, add ¼ cup heavy cream, and boil about 1 minute, or until it thickens to the consistency you prefer. Remove the sauce from the heat and whisk in 2 tablespoons of Dijon mustard, 1 tablespoon of minced chives, and salt and pepper to taste. Pour the sauce over the chicken parts assembled on a serving platter or reserve on the side for individual servings.

Chicken Broth

Makes: 2 quarts Prep time: 12 minutes Cook time: 2½ hours
- 4 roasted chicken carcasses
- 2 yellow onions, roughly chopped
- 2 large carrots, roughly chopped
- 2 celery ribs, roughly chopped
- 1 teaspoon black peppercorn
- 1 bay leaf
- 6 sprigs flat-leaf parsley
- 4 quarts water

1.Combine all of the ingredients in a large stock pot. Bring to a boil, then drop the heat to a medium simmer.

2.Cook for 2½ hours, or until the stock is tasty and well-rounded, and no longer watery. Store in pint or quart containers in the freezer and use it when needed as a base for sauces.

Chicken Livers

Serve these livers with Caramelized Onions if you like. Use a fortified wine such as Madeira, port, sherry, or Marsala.

Makes: 2 servings Prep time: 5 minutes Cook time: 5–7 minutes
- 4 tablespoons butter
- ½ pound chicken livers
- 4 sprigs thyme
- ¼ cup fortified wine
- ½ cup flat-leaf parsley leaves
- sea salt, to taste

1.Heat butter over medium-high in a large frying pan. Once the butter starts foaming, add the salt and chicken livers to the pan and cook for 2 minutes, allowing them to caramelize.

2.Turn the livers over, add the thyme, and cook for an additional minute. Then place the livers on a paper towel–lined plate.

3.Add the fortified wine to the pan, heating just enough to evaporate the alcohol. Stir, removing any cara¬melized bits on the bottom of the pan, 1 to 2 minutes. When the alcohol is gone, it will no longer burn your nose to smell it. Add salt if needed. Return the livers to the pan to coat with sauce. Garnish with parsley.

Pork Belly

Pork belly goes great with Chimichurri sauce.

Makes: 4 servings Prep time: 15 minutes active, 12 hours total Cook time: 1½–2 hours

- 4–5 pound piece pork belly
- 2 tablespoons olive oil
- 4 cups water
- sea salt, to taste

1.Place pork on a sheet pan and season generously with salt, then let sit at least 12 hours in the refrigera¬tor after salting, rotating the pork every few hours so the salt is evenly distributed.

2.Preheat oven to 350°F. Set pork belly skin side up on a wire rack set inside a rimmed baking sheet pan. Pour the water into the baking sheet under the pork.

3.Dry the pork skin with a paper towel. Rub the pork skin with oil and season with more salt. Roast for 1½ to 1¾ hours, adding more water to pan as needed, until the skin is golden brown and a thermometer inserted into thickest part reads 195°F to 200°F.

Lamb Meatballs

Makes: 4–5 servings Prep time: 15 minutes Cook time: 10 minutes

- 1 pound ground lamb
- ½ teaspoon ground cumin
- ½ teaspoon ground coriander
- 4 tablespoons fresh cilantro, finely chopped, plus more to serve
- 2 cloves garlic, minced
- 1½ teaspoons salt
- 1 teaspoon paprika
- ½ teaspoon cayenne pepper, or to taste
- 4 tablespoons olive oil

1.In a large bowl, combine all ingredients except the oil, and mix until the spices are well incorporated.

2.Shape lamb mixture into medium-sized meatballs, about 1½ inches in diameter. Brush them with oil to grill or broil, or pan fry them in a little oil until well browned all over.

3.Serve with more cilantro, if desired.

Brick Chicken

Makes: 2 servings Prep time: 5 minutes active, 45 minutes total Cook time: 25–30 minutes

- 4 chicken thighs, deboned
- 1 tablespoon olive oil
- 5–6 sprigs fresh thyme
- ½ tablespoon unsalted butter
- 1 clove garlic, crushed, with skin on sea salt and freshly ground black pepper, to taste

1.Rinse the chicken thighs and pat them dry. Refrigerate uncovered, skin side up, for at least 30 minutes to dry out the skin.

2.Season the chicken with salt and pepper on both sides and place on a paper towel–lined tray for 15 minutes.

3.Heat a large cast iron or nonstick skillet over medium heat and add the oil. Lay all of the chicken thighs in the skillet, skin side down. It's okay if they overlap. Wrap a slightly smaller skillet with foil and place on top of the chicken (this will act as the "brick"), placing 3 to 4 heavy cans in the skillet to weigh it down.

4.Cook the chicken 3 to 5 minutes, then remove the top skillet and check the skin; adjust the heat and rotate the pan as needed so the skin browns evenly. Replace the top skillet and continue to cook until the skin is golden and crisp and the chicken is cooked about three-quarters of the way through, 10 to 12 more minutes.

5.Add the thyme sprigs, butter, and crushed garlic clove. Remove the top skillet and carefully flip the chicken. Cook, uncovered, until the chicken is cooked through, 4 to 6 more minutes. Transfer to a cutting board and let rest 5 minutes. Cut each piece in half to serve.

Pulled Pork

Makes: 6 servings Prep time: 20 minutes active, 12–24 hours total Cook time: 5-6 hours

- 1 cup peeled, roughly chopped ginger
- 1 cup chopped yellow onion
- 3 tablespoons paprika
- 1 tablespoon Dijon mustard
- ½ cup coarse salt
- ¾ cup peeled cloves garlic
- 1 (5- to 7-pound) pork roast, preferably shoulder or Boston butt
- 6 crisp romaine lettuce leaves
- Pickled Red Onions, to garnish

1.In a blender, blend the ginger, onion, paprika, Dijon mustard, salt, and garlic into a puree. Place the pork into a plastic bag and pour the mixture over the pork; marinate for 12 hours or overnight in the refrigerator. If you can, shift the pork around every few hours to make sure that the marinade is evenly distributed.

2.Preheat the oven to 275°F. Put the pork in a roasting pan and bake for about 5 hours, until it's falling apart and a thermometer inserted into the thickest part reads 170°F.

3.Remove the pork roast from the oven and transfer to a large platter, being careful to save the juices. Allow the meat to rest for about 30 minutes.

4.While still warm, take two forks and shred the meat. Put the shredded pork in a bowl. Pour one quarter of the juice on the shredded pork and mix well to coat. Taste, then add more juice as needed for desired flavor.

5.To serve, spoon the pulled pork mixture onto crisp romaine lettuce leaves. Garnish with pickled onions if you like.

Baked Mackerel

Pair mackerel with Sauce Gribiche or Pickled Red Onions.

Makes: 2 servings Prep time: 10 minutes active, 20 minutes total Cook time: 15 minutes

- 2 mackerel fillets, bones removed
- ¼ cup sea salt
- 1 tablespoon lemon zest
- 2 tablespoons olive oil

1.Preheat oven to 200°F.

2.Combine the sea salt and lemon in a small bowl. Mix well.

3.Season the mackerel filets using a generous amount of the salt mixture on both sides. Let the seasoned fish sit at room temperature for 10 minutes. Afterward, gently scrape the fish and discard the salt mixture.

4.Lightly brush a sheet pan with olive oil and place the fish, skin side down, on the pan. Roast in oven for 15 minutes or until cooked through; the flesh will no longer be translucent. Fish is delicate, and you're more likely to overcook than undercook it.

Chicken Curry

Makes: 4 servings Prep time: 30 minutes Cook time: 15–20 minutes

- 2 pounds boneless, skinless chicken breasts or thighs, cut into 1-inch cubes
- 1½ tablespoons sea salt
- 2½ teaspoons mild curry powder
- 2 tablespoons coconut or olive oil
- 1 (14-ounce) can full-fat coconut milk
- 1 (2½-inch) piece ginger, peeled and sliced
- 4 cloves garlic
- ½ medium onion, chopped
- 2 cups broccoli florets
- 4 cups baby spinach leaves
- zest of 1 lime
- cilantro leaves with tender stems, to garnish

1.Toss the chicken with salt in a medium bowl and let sit for 10 minutes, then add curry powder. Meanwhile, purée the coconut milk, ginger, and garlic in a blender until very smooth.

2.Heat the oil in a large skillet over medium-high heat. Add the onion and stir until softened, about 4 minutes.

3.Add the chicken and the coconut milk mixture to skillet and cook, tossing occasionally, until chicken is cooked through and sauce has thickened, 7 to 10 minutes.

4.Add broccoli florets to the skillet and cook until bright green in color, about 1 minute, then add the spin¬ach and the lime zest. Top with cilantro.

Caramelized Onions

Caramelized onions are a great topping to many foods—I find them especially good on chicken, steak, or hummus.

Makes: 6 servings Prep time: 5 minutes Cook time: 45 minutes

- 4 tablespoons olive oil
- 2 large sweet yellow onions, cut into ¼-inch strips
- 1 cup water, divided
- sea salt, to taste

1.Heat the oil in pan over medium heat and add the cut onions, mixing well to coat them with the oil. Cover the pan with a lid.

2.Once the onions begin to soften, about 2 minutes, add ½ cup of the water and continue cooking on high heat with the lid on. Stir every 3 minutes. When the onions are cooked through, turn the heat down to medium and remove the lid.

3.Allow the onions to caramelize while constantly stirring them; if they get too dark or begin to burn, add a little more water and stir again. The process should take 30 to 40 minutes. Once the onions are brown deep in color, add salt to taste.

Cauliflower Soup

Makes: 3 servings Prep time: 15 minutes Cook time: 20 minutes

- 1½ cups olive oil, divided
- ½ head of cauliflower, cut into ½-inch pieces
- 1 clove garlic, minced
- 1 small shallot, minced
- 1-3 cups water, divided
- sherry vinegar, to taste (optional)
- sea salt, to taste

1.Heat ½ cup of the oil in a frying pan over medium heat. Once the oil is hot, add the cauliflower and sea¬son with salt, cooking until it is light brown, about 5 minutes.

2.Remove the cauliflower and set aside, leaving the oil in the pan. Add garlic to the warm oil and cook until it is golden brown, less than 1 minute, then add the shallots and a little salt, stirring frequently until the shallots are soft, 1 to 2 minutes.

3.Add the cauliflower back to the pan along with 1 cup of the water and cover with a lid. Cook the mixture until the cauliflower is soft, 7 to 8 minutes. If the liquid evaporates before the cauliflower is soft, add more water, ½ cup at a time, to finish cooking.

4. Transfer cauliflower to a blender. Blend at a slow speed, adding the remaining olive oil at a slow drizzle while the blender is on. Once all the oil has been mixed into the soup, blend on high until smooth. Turn blender off, taste, and add salt if needed. Just before serving, add a dash of sherry vinegar to finish off the soup, if desired.

Mushroom Cream Soup

Makes: 4 servings Prep time: 15 minutes Cook time: 30 minutes

- 4 cloves garlic, minced
- 1 cup minced yellow onion
- ¼ cup butter
- 2 pounds cremini and shiitake mushrooms, cut into strips
- ½ cup dry white wine
- 1 cup chicken stock
- 2½ cups whole milk
- 2½ cups heavy cream
- 5 sprigs fresh thyme
- 1 bay leaf
- sea salt, to taste

1. In a medium, heavy-bottomed pot, cook the garlic and onions in the butter over medium-low heat until the onions are translucent, then add mushrooms and salt, and cook for 5 minutes.

2. Continue cooking until all of the juices have been cooked out, then add the wine and cook until the alco¬hol has boiled off (approximately 2 minutes; the liquid should smell good and should not burn your nose).

3. Add the chicken stock, cooking it down by half, 10 to 12 minutes. Then, add the milk and cream, along with the thyme and bay leaf, and lower the heat to medium-low heat. Simmer the soup for 10 minutes while stirring, until all the flavors come together.

4. Strain the soup to separate the onion, garlic, mushrooms, and herbs from the liquid, reserving the liquid. Add the vegetables to a blender with a small amount of the liquid. Blend until smooth, adding the liquid a little at a time until all the liquid is incorporated, and serve.

Creamed Spinach

Makes: 2 servings Prep time: 10 minutes Cook time: 20–25 minutes

- 6 cups fresh, cleaned, and dried spinach leaves
- 3 tablespoons unsalted butter
- 2 tablespoons olive oil
- 1 small sweet onion, minced
- 3 cloves garlic, minced
- ¾ cup heavy cream
- ¼ cup grated Parmesan cheese

- sea salt, to taste
- freshly ground black pepper, to taste

1.Bring a medium pot of water to a boil over high heat. Blanch the spinach for 10 to 15 seconds in salted water and then place in an ice water bath for 30 seconds. Drain, and squeeze out the excess water. Chop the cooked spinach into small pieces.

2.Heat the butter and oil in a large skillet over medium-high heat and add the minced onion and garlic. Cook, stirring frequently, until soft, 3 to 4 minutes.

3.Add the cream and cook until it reduces by half, about 10 minutes. Then add the Parmesan and season with salt and pepper to taste, stirring frequently until the cheese has melted. Add spinach and cook until it's hot, about 5 more minutes. Serve immediately.

Cauliflower Mash

Makes: 4 servings Prep time: 12 minutes Cook time: 6 minutes

- 1 head cauliflower
- 2 tablespoons olive oil
- 1 clove garlic, minced
- 2 tablespoons chopped fresh rosemary
- 2 tablespoons butter
- 2 tablespoons heavy cream
- sea salt, to taste

1.Prepare a steamer basket over 4 inches of water in a pot, and bring to a boil. Break the cauliflower into florets and add them to the steamer basket over the boiling water. Allow to steam for 1 minute uncovered, then cover the pot and steam until soft, about 3 minutes more.

2.Heat olive oil in a skillet over medium-low heat and add chopped rosemary and garlic, cooking 1 to 2 minutes. Add butter and melt, and add cauliflower to coat with seasoning. Cook 1 more minute.

3.Mash cauliflower with a potato masher in the skillet. Pour contents of skillet into blender, and add heavy cream while blending. Add salt while blending. Serve like mashed potatoes.

Roasted Cauliflower

A common mistake when roasting cauliflower is to not roast it long enough; a longer roast will produce more caramelization and a tastier end product. For the same reason, do not move the florets during the cooking process. Serve with Tahini Dressing, if you'd like.

Makes: 2 servings Prep time: 8 minutes Cook time: 45 minutes

- 1 head cauliflower
- 4 tablespoons olive oil
- sea salt, to taste

1.Preheat oven to 375°F.

2.Break the cauliflower into florets and toss in a large mixing bowl with olive oil and salt.

3.Spread on a baking sheet and bake in the oven for 30 to 45 minutes, or until well caramelized.

Spicy Variation: Add the following into the mixing bowl when coating the cauliflower with oil: 2 tablespoons minced garlic, 1 teaspoon cumin, 1 teaspoon paprika, ½ teaspoon turmeric, and ¼ teaspoon cayenne pepper.

Pesto

In my opinion, pesto goes well on just about anything, especially noodles (including no-carb shirataki noo¬dles), fish, and chicken. It brings a bright, fresh, basil flavor to your dish. You can store pesto in a clean ice cube tray and defrost individual cubes when you want to use them.

Makes: 4–6 servings Prep time: 15 minutes

- 4 loosely packed cups fresh basil leaves
- ½ cup grated Parmesan cheese
- ⅓ cup pine nuts or walnuts
- 3 cloves garlic, minced
- ¾ cup olive oil, plus more as needed
- sea salt, to taste
- freshly ground black pepper, to taste

1.Pulse basil and nuts in a food processor until homogeneous. Add the cheese and garlic, and pulse until combined.

2.Slowly drizzle in the olive oil while the processor is running on low speed if your machine has multiple speeds, otherwise, add 1 to 2 tablespoons of oil at a time and check consistency before adding more. Once the oil is completely combined and the pesto is the consistency you want, mix in the salt and pepper.

Scott J. Barnard

CONCLUSION

So with all of the information I have provided you in this book, I wish you luck in your journey to a healthy weight and to a body that is healed from whatever ails you.

No more deprivation diets of fat-free, man-made foods ... You need real food, real satisfaction, and a healthy mind and body.

AUTHOR BIO

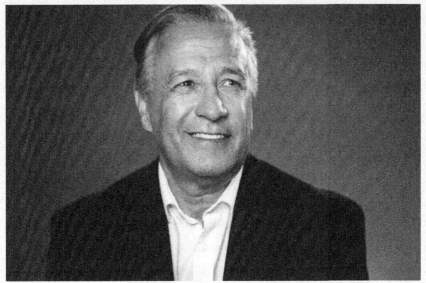

SCOTT J. BARNARD

Scott J. Barnard is an author and medical expert with years of experience as a GP and health consultant. He has worked for countless years in the medical field, dealing with patients and working with the cardiovascular system, immune system, respiratory system, and more.

Scott has personally trained hundreds of students through courses and face-to-face, and he's coached countless more to help them pass their medical exams and break into the field. Armed with a wide range of knowledge, he has helped his students become doctors, nurses, paramedics, physicians, and more.

With his book, *Medical Terminology for Health Professions 4.0*, he hopes to inspire and empower a new wave of medical students to reach the next level by passing their exams and succeeding in their careers.

Scott has condensed his knowledge and research into a comprehensive list of terminology which will help students understand, pronounce, and memorize thousands of medical terms.

Scott J. Barnard is the author of several books, including:
- MEDICAL TERMINOLOGY FOR HEALTH PROFESSIONS 4.0
- THE METABOLIC APPROACH TO OBESITY 4.0
- THYROID SYMPTOMS 4.0
- ANTI-INFLAMMATORY HERBAL HEALING 4.0
- REVERSING YOUR CHILD'S EATING DISORDER 4.0

LinkedIn: www.linkedin.com/in/scottjbarnard/
email: scottbarnard1959@gmail.com

Thank you for reading this book.

If you enjoyed it please visit the site where you purchased it and write a brief review. Your feedback is important to me and will help other readers decide whether to read the book too.

Thank you!

Scott J.Barnard

Do you want more?
Grab "Reversing Your Child's Eating Disorder 4.0" for free

Instructions

Scan the Qr code or click on the link and click BUY NOW, click on Add a Coupon and enter this coupon that gives you the **100% discount code**

BY2HZUA5ZD

Now Download the book for Free

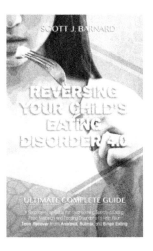

So don't wait! This is the book for you!

https://mgdluxurybooks.com/b/8x0rK

BONUS

Download **FREE** and listen to the audiobook "The Metabolic Approach to Obesity 4.0"wherever you are.

You will download the audiobook in MP3 format and divided by chapters.

Instructions

Scan the Qr code or click on the link and click BUY NOW, click on Add a Coupon and enter this coupon that gives you the **100% discount code**

0Z29520BPJ

Now Download the audiobook for Free

https://mgdluxurybooks.com/b/ZO0oK

Printed in Great Britain
by Amazon

36113188R00126